MW01234801

KETO BREAD

50 BEST LOW-CARB BREAD RECIPES

Doc Julian

The following eBook is reproduced below with the goal of

providing information that is as accurate and reliable as possible.

Regardless, purchasing this eBook can be seen as consent to the fact that both the publisher and the author of this book are in no way experts on the topics discussed within and that any recommendations or suggestions that are made herein are for entertainment purposes only. Professionals should be consulted as needed prior to undertaking any of the action endorsed herein.

This declaration is deemed fair and valid by both the American Bar Association and the Committee of Publishers Association and is legally binding throughout the United States.

Furthermore, the transmission, duplication, or reproduction of any of the following work including specific information will be considered an illegal act irrespective of if it is done electronically or in print.

This extends to creating a secondary or tertiary copy of the work or a recorded copy and is only allowed with the express written consent from the Publisher. All additional rights reserved.

The information in the following pages is broadly considered a truthful and accurate account of facts and as such, any inattention, use, or misuse of the information in question by the reader will render any resulting actions solely under their purview.

There are no scenarios in which the publisher or the original author of this work can be in any fashion deemed liable for any hardship or damages that may befall them after undertaking information described herein.

Additionally, the information in the following pages is intended only for informational purposes and should thus be thought of as universal. As befitting its nature, it is presented without assurance regarding its prolonged validity or interim quality.

Trademarks that are mentioned are done without written consent and can in no way be considered an endorsement from the trademark holder.

Table of Contents

20. Coconut Flour Pizza Crust

21. Mini Paleo Pizza Bases Crusts

22. Keto Zucchini Bread with Walnut Crust

23. Keto Pumpkin Bread

24. Low Carb Blueberry English Muffin Bread Loaf

25. Cinnamon Almond Flour Bread

26. Keto Chocolate Zucchini Bread

27. Low Carb Gluten Free Cranberry Bread

28. Coconut Flour Psyllium Husk Bread

29. Cheesy Keto Garlic Bread - Using Mozzarella Dough

30. Nut-Free Keto Bread

31. Keto Coconut Flour Flatbread

32. Homemade Nut and Seed Keto Bread

33. Cinnamon & Honey Keto Bread

34. Cheesy Skillet Bread

35. Keto Low Carb Banana Bread

36. Keto Fathead Rolls

37. Keto Cinnamon Cloud Bread

38. Keto Bread Rolls

39. Easy Oopsie Flatbread

40. Keto Pumpkin Chia Muffins

41. Keto Mozzarella Dough Bagels

42. Keto Low Carb Naan Bread

43. Sourdough Keto Baguettes

44. Keto Pumpkin Bread French Toast

45. 90 Second Bread

INTRODUCTION

I want to thank you and congratulate you for Downloading the book, " *KETO BREAD - 50 BEST LOW-CARB BREAD RECIPES*

Studies have demonstrated that a higher protein, low carbohydrate diet promotes superior results for fat loss, improvements in blood lipid parameters and increased thermogenesis in individuals with obesity and insulin resistance and may help to resolve the metabolic blocks that can prevent fat loss.

The general dietary guidelines involve avoidance of high carbohydrate foods such as bread, pasta, potatoes, rice etc. as well as all simple carbohydrates such as sugar, honey and fruit juice.

Protein is included in every meal as this helps to reduce appetite, regulate blood glucose levels and preserve lean muscle mass. Examples of protein foods are fish, chicken, turkey, meat, eggs, cheese, tofu and tempeh.

Protein drinks such as whey protein isolate or soy protein may be utilized. Soy protein is especially beneficial as it has been shown to stimulate thyroid hormone production, reduce fat levels and promote fat loss, due to the phytoestrogens and essential fatty acids it contains.

Adequate fat intake is also essential as this enhances fat burning by the body while reducing synthesis of fatty acids in the body which both promote fat loss. Optimal sources of fats are flaxseed oil, fish oil, avocado, olive oil, nuts and seeds.

To provide balanced nutrition, vitamins, minerals, and fiber and to promote detoxification it is also essential to consume

3-4 cups of low carbohydrate vegetables or salad daily with one optional serve of fresh fruit daily.

When beginning a Ketogenic diet program some discomfort may be experienced such as headaches, irritability, fatigue and hunger for the first 2-7 days, however thereafter it is very easy to adhere to the diet and it actually reduces appetite, carbohydrate cravings and increases energy levels.

The Ketogenic diet produces very good results when followed consistently. Long term success is more likely if a holistic attitude is adopted that addresses diet, exercise, nutritional supplements and psychological factors as well as any specific health challenges that are unique to the individual.

When the ideal body fat percentage is achieved the diet may be gradually adjusted to include more complex carbohydrates such as whole grains, starchy vegetables and fruit while as much as possible avoiding all other simple carbohydrates such as sugar, honey and refined flours. Simultaneously it is essential to ensure that protein is included in every meal.

This more relaxed type of dietary approach can be maintained indefinitely in conjunction with a regular exercise program to ensure that body weight and composition remains stable.

This COMPLETE GUIDE comprising of 50 quick and delicious keto bread recipes is an absolute must have for all families, carers and associated professionals who need a thorough understanding of the Ketogenic Diet and it's application for helping reduce weight gain and some other health conditions.

Thanks again for reading this book, I hope you enjoy it!

CHAPTER 1

What Does A Ketogenic Diet Look Like?

When the average person eats a meal rich in carbs, their body takes those carbs and converts them into glucose for fuel. Glucose is the body's main source of fuel when carbs are present in the body, on a Keto diet there are very low if any at all carbs consumed which forces the body to utilize other forms of energy to keep the body functioning properly.

This is where healthy fats come into play, with the absence of carbs the liver takes fatty acids in the body and converts them into ketone bodies.

An ideal Keto diet should consist of:

• 70-80% Fat

• 20-25% Protein

• 5-10% Carbs

You should not be eating more than 20g of carbs per day to maintain the typical Ketogenic diet. I personally ate less than 10g per day for a more drastic experience but I achieved my initial goals and then some. I lost 28 lbs. in a little under 3 weeks.

When the body is fueled completely by fat it enters a state called "Ketosis," which is a natural state for the body. After all of the sugars and unhealthy fats have been removed from the body during the first couple of weeks, the body is now free run on healthy fats.

Ketosis has many potential benefits-related to rapid weight loss, health or performance. In certain situations like type 1 diabetes excessive ketosis can become extremely dangerous, where as in certain cases paired with intermittent fasting can be extremely beneficial for people suffering from type 2 diabetes.

Ketogenic diet are extreme low-carb diets where the aim is to be in a state of ketosis, meaning that the body is burning fat as fuel as opposed to glucose.

This state is achieved, largely, by simply depriving the body of glucose via the food source is available through the dieters nutritional plan.

Being in ketosis allows the body to process fat and use it as fuel in a way that no other state allows as easily. Carbohydrates are much easier to convert and use as fuel, so when you are providing plenty of these to your body, you need to burn and use all of those before your body will finally begin converting and using fat as fuel.

Another benefit of being in a state of ketosis is that excess ketones are not harmful to your system in any way whatsoever. Any key tones that you create which are not needed by your body are simply excreted through urine, easily and harmlessly.

In fact, this excellent benefit is the reason why you can check whether you are in a state of ketosis using urine testing strips in the morning.

When your body gets used to being in ketosis, it will actually begin to prefer ketones to glucose. This is the ideal state that you want your body to be in - no longer craving sugar whatsoever, and in fact preferring protein as a fuel source as opposed to sugar.

For someone new to Keto, it can be very challenging to stick to a low-carb diet, even though fat is the cornerstone of this diet you should not be eating any and all kinds of fat. Healthy fats are essential, but what is healthy fat you might ask.

CHAPTER 2

50 Keto Low Carb Bread Recipes

1. Keto Bread with Collagen

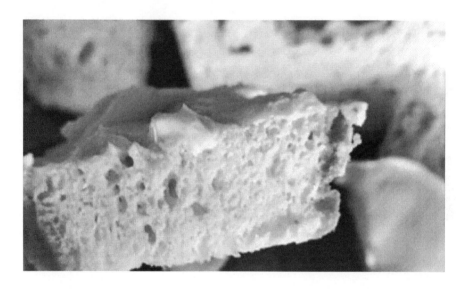

Keto Collagen Bread is a zero Net Carbs Per Slice. It's also Bulletproof and Paleo - which means it's dairy free, grain free, gluten free and it uses heat stable collagen protein.

Grass-fed hydrolyzed collagen protein is reported to help support healthy skin, hair, nails, joints, gut health and anti-aging just to name a few of its many benefits.

This bread is fluffy, delicious, not too eggy and all this with no carbs per slice. The loaf is standard size and sliced into 12 generous slices.

You can easily up the fat content when consuming this bread simply by adding a big slather of ghee or butter, but the possibilities are endless.

Prep Time : 10 min

Cook Time: 40 min

Total Time: 50 min

Nutrition Facts (per 100g)

- Energy - 203 kcal
- Total Fat - 16g
- Fat Percentage - 69%
- Net Carbohydrates - 1,7g
- Protein - 8g

Note: 10g butter per 50g bread makes the fat percentage 82%

Ingredients

30g coconut flour

35g ground flaxseed

25g psyllium husk powder

25g oat fiber (Nu Naturals Oat Fiber)

20g hydrolyzed collagen (Iconfit)

2g xanthan gum

2g guarkum (4g one of them is enough too)

4g pink salt

6g baking powder

Dried ginger powder and cardamon to taste

80g seedes (sesame, sunflower, pumpkin and Hemp Hearts) 1 spl (apple) cider vinegar

2 eggs

200g hot water (50C)

Instructions:

Step 1 - Preheat the oven to 170C (160C fan).

Step 2 - Mix all dry ingredients together, then mix in eggs and apple cider vinegar.

Step 3 - Finally add hot water and mix into even dough.

Step 4 - Devide the dough between preferred bread forms and garnish with sesame seeds. I used 4 small ones this time.

Step 5 - Bake for 40-60 minutes, depending on the size of the forms.

Step 6 - Serve with butter.

2. KETO ALMND FLUR BRD

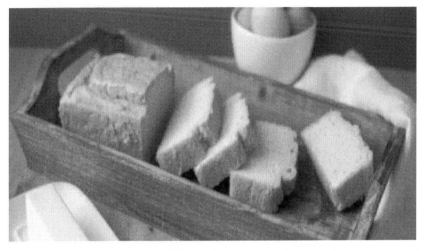

This recipe contains psyllium husks. Psyllium does not only help with the texture, but also makes your entirely grain free loaf taste a bit like whole-wheat bread. Last but not least, psyllium is a fantastic source of fibre.

There's one more secret ingredient that helps this bread have a texture that resembles regular bread: xanthan gum. Low carb bread lacks the gluten which occurs in wheat, which can make it crumbly. The xanthan gum gives grain free bread a stronger structure and a better crust.

- Prep Time - 5 minutes

- Cook Time - 45 minutes
- Total Time - 50 minutes

Nutrition Facts

Fat - 14.2g22%

Carbohydrates - 4.1g1%

Fiber - 3.5g15%

Sugar - 0.7g1%

Protein - 5.7g11%

Ingredients

1 1/2 Cup Almond Flour

6 Large eggs Separated

1/4 cup Butter melted

3 tsp Baking powder

1/4 tsp Cream of Tartar It's ok if you don't have this

1 pinch Pink Himalayan Salt

6 drops Liquid Stevia optional

Instructions

Preheat oven to 375.

Separate the egg whites from the yolks. Add Cream of Tartar to the whites and beat until soft peaks are achieved.

In a food processor combine the egg yolks, 1/3 of the beaten egg whites, melted butter, almond flour, baking powder and salt (Adding ~6 drops of liquid stevia to the batter can help reduce the mild egg taste). Mix until combined. This will be a lumpy thick dough until the whites are added.

Add the remaining 2/3 of the egg whites and gently process until fully incorporated. Be careful not to overmix as this is what gives the bread it's volume!

Pour mixture into a buttered 8x4 loaf pan. Bake for 30 minutes.

Check with a toothpick to ensure the bread is cooked through. Enjoy! 1 loaf makes 20 slices.

3. KETO LOW CARB COCONUT FLOUR BRD

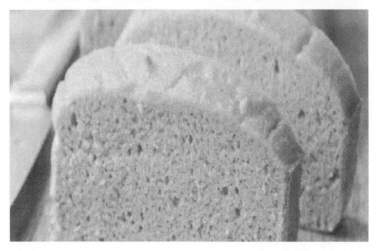

Keto low carb coconut bread is a fantastic substitute for my regular keto bread but it is is nut free, gluten free and slightly lower in calories. The bread is fluffy, sliceable and totally delicious.

Prep Time - 10 minutes

Cook Time - 50 minutes

Total Time - 1 hour 30 minutes

Nutrition Facts

Calories 95 - Calories from Fat : 81%

Fat:9g - 14%

Saturated Fat:5g - 31%

Cholesterol:97mg - 32%

Sodium 117mg - 5%

Potassium 32mg - 1%

Carbohydrates 1g - 0%

Fiber 1g - 4%

Sugar 0.2g - 0%

Protein 3g - 6%

Vitamin A 300IU - 6%

Calcium 10mg - 1%

Iron 0.7mg - 4%

Ingredients

- 7 Large Eggs
- 1/2 cup Coconut Flour 40g / 1.2 oz
- 1/2 cup Butter 120g / 4 oz (use 1/2 cup olive/coconut oil for dairy free)
- 1/4 tsp Salt
- 1/4 tsp baking powder (aluminium free if possible)
- 1/2 tsp xanthan gum (optional)

Directions

Preheat oven to 180 C (355 F).

Crack the eggs into a bowl and mix for 1 minute until well combined.

Add the coconut flour, butter, salt, baking powder and xanthan gum, and mix until completely combined. The mixture will become quite thick.

Line an 8.5 X 5-inch (21.5 x 12.7 cm) loaf tin with parchment paper and pour the batter into the tin. Level the top with a spatula if uneven.

Bake for 50 minutes or until a skewer comes out of the middle clean.

Nutrition information is for 1 slice. Slice and store in the fridge for up to 5 days or in the freezer for up to 2 weeks. This bread freezes well.

4. DIR-FR KETO CLUD BRD

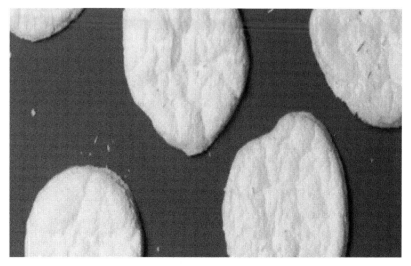

Light and fluffy Oopsie Rolls or Cloud Bread makes a great sandwich bread replacement. Ultra low carb, keto, grain free and gluten free.

Prep Time - 10 mins

Cook Time - 30 mins

Total Time - 40 mins

Nutrition Facts

- Calories: 87
- Protein: 5g

- Fat: 7g

- Carbs: .6g

- Fiber: 0g

- Net Carbs: .6g

Ingredients

3 eggs

3 tbsp coconut cream spoon from refrigerated can of full-fat coconut milk

1/2 tsp baking powder

optional toppings: sea salt black pepper and rosemary or whatever seasonings you like!

Instructions

Firstly, prep everything. Once you start going, you'll need to move quickly so have everything handy. Pre-heat the oven to 325f degrees and arrange a rack in the middle. Line a baking sheet with parchment paper and set aside.

Grab your tools: hand mixer (you can use a stand mixer, but I find it to be better for whipping egg whites so I can stay in control), all ingredients, any additional seasonings, two mixing bowls (the larger one should be used for egg whites), a large spoon to scoop and drop the bread with.

Using a full-fat can of coconut milk that has been refrigerated overnight or several hours, spoon out the top coconut cream and add to the smaller bowl.

Separate eggs into the two bowls, adding the yolk to the bowl with the cream and be careful to not let the yolk get into the whites in the larger bowl.

Using a hand mixer, beat the yolk and cream together first until nice and creamy, make sure there are no clumps of coconut left.

Wash your whisks well and dry them.Add the baking powder into the whites and start beating on medium with the hand mixer for a few minutes, moving around and you'll see it get firmer. Keep going for a few minutes, you want to get it as thick as you can with stiff peaks. The thicker the better. Just don't over-do it.

Once you can stop and dip the whisks in leaving peaks behind, you're ready.Quickly and carefully add the yolk-coconut mixture into the whites, folding with a spatula, careful not to deflate too much. Keep going until everything is well combined but still fluffy.

Now you can grab your spoon and start dropping your batter down on the baking sheet. Keep going as quickly and carefully as you can, or it will start to melt. They should look pillow-y.

Steadily add your baking sheet to the middle rack in the oven and bake for approx. 20-25 minutes. You should be able to scoop them up with your spatula and see a fluffy top and a flat bottom. Store in the fridge for about a week or freeze.

5. LOW CARB KETO MDMI NUT BRD

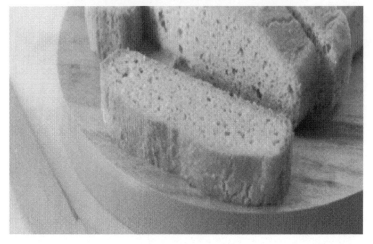

Unlike many low carb bread recipes that turn out very dense and eggy products, this one uses xanthan gum to achieve a softer texture that resembles the gluten in regular wheat bread. It's hard to believe that one slice has only 1.8g of net carbs.

Prep Time - 5 minutes

Cook Time - 30-40 minutes

Nutrition Facts (per slice):

Calories: 173

Fat: 15g (78%)

Carbohydrates: 3.5g (8%)

Fiber: 1.7g

Net Carbohydrates: 1.8g

Protein: 6g (14%)

Ingredients

5 oz macadamia nuts I used the Royal Hawaiian brand

5 large eggs

1/4 cup coconut flour (28 g)

1/2 teaspoon baking soda

1/2 teaspoon apple cider vinegar

Instructions

Preheat oven to 350F.

To a blender or food processor, add macadamia nuts and pulse until it becomes a nut butter. If your blender does not do a good job without liquid, add in eggs one at a time until the consistency is that of a nut butter.

Scrape down sides of blender or food processor, and add in remaining eggs. Blend until well-incorporated.

Add in coconut flour, baking soda and apple cider vinegar and pulse until incorporated.

Grease a standard-size bread pan and add in batter. Smooth surface of batter and place on bottom rack of oven for 30-40 minutes, or until the top is golden brown.

Remove from oven and allow to cool in pan for 15-20 minutes before removing.

Will store in an air-tight container at room temperature for 3-4 days at room temperature, or for one week in the fridge.

6. KETO FI BRD WITH GARLIC AND HRBS

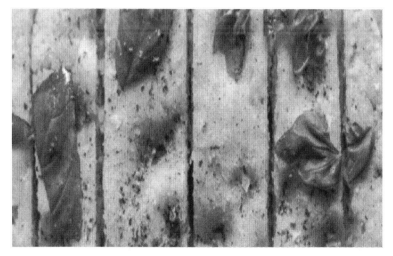

Prep Time: 15 minutes

Cook Time: 20 minutes

Total Time: 35 minutes

Nutrition Facts:

- Calories: 352
- Fat: 29.3g
- Net carbs: 4.3g (total carbs: 6.7g, dietary fiber: 2.4g)
- Protein: 16.4g

Ingredients

Dry Ingredients

   1 cup Almond Flour

   ¼ cup Coconut Flour

   ½ tsp Xanthan Gum

   1 tsp Garlic Powder

   1 tsp Flaky Salt

   ½ tsp Baking Soda

   ½ tsp Baking Powder

Wet Ingredients

   2 eggs

   1 tbsp Lemon Juice

   2 tsp Olive oil + 2 tbsp Olive Oil to drizzle

Instructions

Heat oven to 350 and line a baking tray or 8-inch round pan with parchment.

Whisk together the dry ingredients making sure there are no lumps.

Beat the egg, lemon juice, and oil until combined.

Mix the wet and the dry together, working quickly, and scoop the dough into your pan.

Make sure not to mix the wet and dry until you are ready to put the bread in the oven because the leavening reaction begins once it is mixed!!!

Smooth the top and edges with a spatula dipped in water (or your hands) then use your finger to dimple the dough. Don't be afraid to go deep on the dimples! Again, a little water keeps it from sticking.

Bake covered for about 10 minutes. Drizzle with Olive Oil bake for an additional 10-15 minutes uncovering to brown gently.

Top with more flaky salt, olive oil (optional), a dash of Italian seasoning and fresh basil. Let cool completely before slicing for optimal texture!!

7. KETO CULIFLWR BREAD

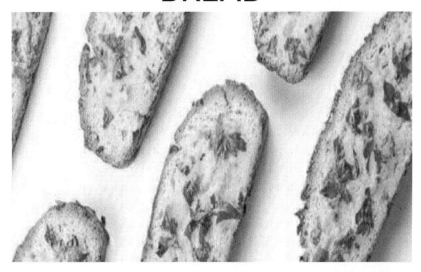

This delicious cauliflower recipe has 3.7 grams of fiber in each slice, which not only lowers your net carb intake but also keeps your digestion running smoothly and your gut bugs happy.

Prep Time: 15 minutes

Total Time: 1 hour and 10 minutes

Nutrition Facts:

- Calories: 142
- Carbohydrates: 6.5g
- Fiber: 3.7g

- Protein: 7.1g

Ingredients

3 cup Cauliflower ("riced" using food processor*)

10 large Egg (separated)

1/4 tsp Cream of tartar (optional)

1 1/4 cup Coconut flour

1 1/2 tbsp Gluten-free baking powder

1 tsp Sea salt

6 tbsp Butter (unsalted, measured solid, then melted; can use ghee for dairy-free)

6 cloves Garlic (minced)

1 tbsp Fresh rosemary (chopped)

1 tbsp Fresh parsley (chopped)

Instructions

Preheat the oven to 350 degrees F (177 degrees C). Line a 9x5 in (23x13 cm) loaf pan with parchment paper.

Steam the riced cauliflower. You can do this in the microwave (cooked for 3-4 minutes, covered in plastic) OR in a steamer basket over water on the stove (line with cheesecloth if the holes in the steamer basket are too big, and steam for a few minutes). Both ways, steam until the cauliflower is soft and tender. Allow the cauliflower to cool enough to handle.

Meanwhile, use a hand mixer to beat the egg whites and cream of tartar until stiff peaks form.

Place the coconut flour, baking powder, sea salt, egg yolks, melted butter, garlic, and 1/4 of the whipped egg whites in a food processor.

When the cauliflower has cooled enough to handle, wrap it in kitchen towel and squeeze several times to release as much moisture as possible. (This is important - the end result should be very dry and clump together.) Add the cauliflower to the food processor.

Process until well combined. (Mixture will be dense and a little crumbly.)

Add the remaining egg whites to the food processor. Fold in just a little, to make it easier to process. Pulse a few times until just incorporated. (Mixture will be fluffy.) Fold in the chopped parsley and rosemary. (Don't overmix to avoid breaking down the egg whites too much.)

Transfer the batter into the lined baking pan. Smooth the top and round slightly. If desired, you can press more herbs into the top (optional).

Bake for about 45-50 minutes, until the top is golden. Cool completely before removing and slicing.

8. 15-MINUTE GLUTN FR, LW CRB & KETO TRTILLS

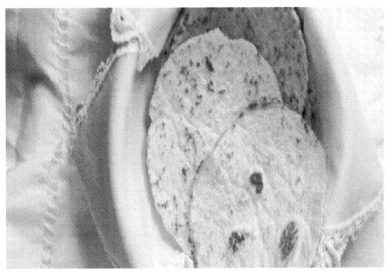

These (15-minute!) gluten free and keto tortillas are super pliable, easy-peasy and make the best low carb tacos... at just 2g net carbs a pop.

Prep Time: 10 minutes

Cook Time: 5 minutes

Total Time: 15 minutes

Nutrition Facts:

Doc Julian

Calories 89 - Calories from Fat 54

Fat 6g - 9%

- Saturated Fat 1g - 5%

Cholesterol 20mg - 7%

Sodium 51mg - 2%

Potassium 58mg - 2%

Carbohydrates 4g - 1%

Fiber 2g - 8%

Protein 3g - 6%

Vitamin A 30IU - 1%

Calcium 50mg - 5%

Iron 0.7mg - 4%

Ingredients

96 g almond flour

24 g coconut flour

2 teaspoons xanthan gum

1 teaspoon baking powder

1/8-1/4 teaspoon kosher salt depending on whether sweet or savory

2 teaspoons apple cider vinegar

1 egg lightly beaten

3 teaspoons water

Instructions

Add almond flour, coconut flour, xanthan gum, baking powder

and salt to food processor. Pulse until thoroughly combined.

Pour in apple cider vinegar with the food processor running. Once it has distributed evenly, pour in the egg. Followed by the water. Stop the food processor once the dough forms into a ball. The dough will be sticky to touch.

Wrap dough in cling film and knead it through the plastic for a minute or two. Think of it a bit like a stress ball. Allow dough to rest for 10 minutes (and up to two days in the fridge).

Heat up a skillet (preferably) or pan over medium heat. You can test the heat by sprinkling a few water droplets, if the drops evaporate immediately your pan is too hot. The droplets should 'run' through the skillet.

Break the dough into eight 1" balls (26g each). Roll out between two sheets of parchment or waxed paper with a rolling pin or using a tortilla press (easier!) until each round is 5-inches in diameter.

Transfer to skillet and cook over medium heat for just 3-6 seconds (very important). Flip it over immediately (using a thin spatula or knife), and continue to cook until just lightly golden on each side (though with the traditional charred marks), 30 to 40 seconds.

The key is not to overcook them, as they will no longer be pliable or puff up. Keep them warm wrapped in kitchen cloth until serving. To rewarm, heat briefly on both sides, until just warm (less than a minute).

9. KETO COCONUT FLUR FLATBREAD

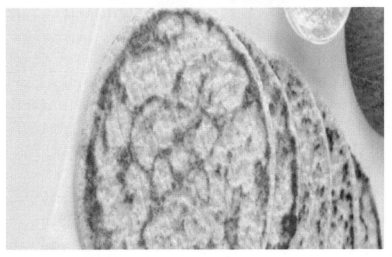

Coconut flour flatbread also known as coconut flour tortillas are easy, soft and flexible keto tortilla with only 2.6 g net carbs per serve.

Prep Time: 10 mins

Cook Time: 5 mins

Total Time: 15 mins

Nutrition Facts:

Calories 66 - Calories from Fat 30

Fat 3.3g - 5%

Carbohydrates 7.3g - 2%

Fiber 4.7g - 20%

Sugar 2g - 2%

Protein 2g - 4%

Ingredients

2 tablespoons psyllium husk (9g)

1/2 cup coconut flour fine, fresh, no lumps (60g)

1 cup lukewarm water (240ml)

1 tablespoon olive oil (15ml)

1/4 teaspoons baking soda

1/4 teaspoons salt - optional

Cooking

1 teaspoon olive oil to rub/oil the non stick pan

Instructions

Make the dough

In a medium mixing bowl, combine the psyllium husk and coconut flour (if lumps are in your flour use a fork to smash them BEFORE measuring the flour, amount must be precise).

Add in the lukewarm water (I used tap water about 40C/bath temperature), olive oil, and baking soda. Give a good stir with a spatula, then use your hands to knead the dough. Add salt now if you want. I never add the salt in contact with baking soda to avoid deactivating the leaving agent.

Knead for 1 minute. The dough is moist and it gets softer and slightly dryer as you go. It should come together easily to form a dough as on my picture. If not, too sticky, add more husk, 1/2 teaspoon at a time, knead for 30 sec and see how it goes. The dough will always be a bit moist but it shouldn't stick to your hands at all. It must come together as a dough.

Set aside 10 minute in the mixing bowl.Now the dough must be soft, elastic and hold well together, it is ready to roll.Roll/shape the flatbread

Cut the dough into 4 even pieces, roll each pieces into a small ball.

Place one of the dough ball between two pieces of parchment paper, press the ball with your hand palm to stick it well to the paper and start rolling with a rolling pin as thin as you like a bread.

Un peel the first layer of parchment paper from your flatbread. Use a lid to cut out round flatbread. Keep the outside dough to reform a ball and roll more flatbread - that is how I make 2 extra flatbread from the 4 balls above!

Cook in non stick pan

Warm a non stick tefal crepe/ pancake pan under medium/high heat- or use any non stick pan of your choice, the one you would use for your pancakes.

Add one teaspoon of olive oil or vegetable oil of your choice onto a piece of absorbent paper. Rub the surface of the pan to make sure it is slightly oiled. Don't leave any drops of oil or the bread will fry!

Flip over the flatbread on the hot pan and peel off carefully the last piece of parchment paper.

Cook for 2-3 minutes on the first side, flip over using a spatula and cook for 1-2 more minute on the other side.

Cool down the flatbread on a plate and use as a sandwich wrap later or enjoy hot as a side dish. I recommend a drizzle of olive oil, crushed garlic and herbs before serving ! (optional but delish!)

Repeat the rolling, cooking for the next 3 flatbread. Make sure you rub the oiled absorbent paper onto the saucepan each time to avoid the bread to stick to the pan.

Store in the pantry in an airtight box or on a plate covered with plastic wrap to keep them soft, for up to 3 days.

Rewarm in the same pan or if you want to give them a little crisp rewarm in the hot oven on a baking sheet for 1-2 minutes at 150C.

10. LOW CARB BAKED CAULIFLOWER TRTILLS

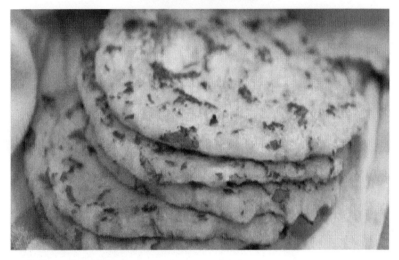

Prep Time: 10 minutes

Cook Time: 17 minutes

Cooling TIme: 15 minutes

Total Time: 27 minutes

Nutrition Facts:

Calories 42 - Calories from Fat 9

Fat 1g - 2%

Saturated Fat 0g - 0%

Cholesterol 62mg - 21%

Sodium 42mg - 2%

Potassium 182mg - 5%

Carbohydrates 3g - 1%

Fiber 1g - 4%

Sugar 1g - 1%

Protein 3g - 6%

Vitamin A 90IU - 2%

Vitamin C 25.7mg - 31%

Calcium 21mg - 2%

Iron 0.5mg - 3%

    Net Carbs 2g

    % Carbs: 27.6%

    % Protein: 41.4%

    % Fat: 31%

Ingredients

    3/4 large head cauliflower (or two cups riced)

    2 large eggs (Vegans, sub flax eggs)

    1/4 cup chopped fresh cilantro

    1/2 medium lime, juiced and zested

    salt & pepper, to taste

Instructions

Preheat the oven to 375 degrees F., and line a baking sheet with parchment paper.

Trim the cauliflower, cut it into small, uniform pieces, and pulse in a food processor in batches until you get a couscous-like consistency. The finely riced cauliflower should make about 2 cups packed.

Place the cauliflower in a microwave-safe bowl and microwave for 2 minutes, then stir and microwave again for another 2 minutes. If you don't use a microwave, a steamer works just as well. Place the cauliflower in a fine cheesecloth or thin dish-towel and squeeze out as much liquid as possible, being careful not to burn yourself. Dishwashing gloves are suggested as it is very hot.

In a medium bowl, whisk the eggs. Add in cauliflower, cilantro, lime, salt and pepper. Mix until well combined. Use your hands to shape 6 small "tortillas" on the parchment paper.

Bake for 10 minutes, carefully flip each tortilla, and return to the oven for an additional 5 to 7 minutes, or until completely set. Place tortillas on a wire rack to cool slightly.

Heat a medium-sized skillet on medium. Place a baked tortilla in the pan, pressing down slightly, and brown for 1 to 2 minutes on each side. Repeat with remaining tortillas.

11. KETO BUTTERY LW CARB FLTBRD

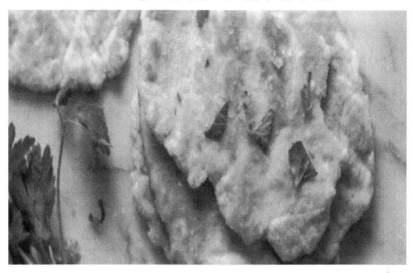

Prep Time: 5 minutes

Cook Time: 2 minutes

Total Time: 7 minutes

Nutrition Facts:

- Calories 232
- Total Fat 19g
- Carbohydrates 9g
- Fiber 5g

- Protein 9g

Ingredients

1 cup Almond Flour

2 tbsp Coconut Flour

2 tsp Xanthan Gum

½ tsp Baking Powder

½ tsp Flake Salt + more to garnish

1 Whole Egg + 1 Egg White

1 tbsp Water

1 tbsp Oil for frying

1 tbsp melted Butter-for slathering

Instructions

Whisk together the dry ingredients (flours, xanthan gum, baking powder, salt) until well combined.

Add the egg and egg white and beat gently into the flour to incorporate. The dough will begin to form.

Add the tablespoon of water and begin to work the dough to allow the flour and xanthan gum to absorb the moisture.

Cut the dough in 4 equal parts and press each section out with cling wrap. Watch the video for instructions!

Heat a large skillet over medium heat and add oil.

Fry each flatbread for about 1 min on each side.

Brush with butter (while hot) and garnish with salt and chopped parsley.

12. FLUFF KT BUNS

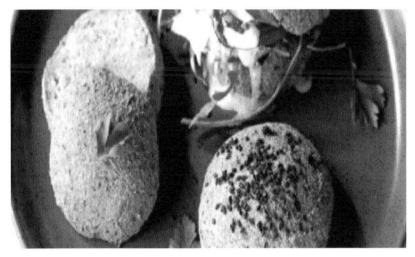

These keto hamburger buns taste just like the real thing — all with no gluten, grains, or nuts. This fiber-rich supplement helps these keto buns rise and allows the dough to stretch without gluten-filled white flour.

With added rise from baking powder and beaten egg whites, these buns are perfectly chewy and fluffy. Since psyllium husk can be harsh on your gut, these rolls are best enjoyed in moderation.

Prep Time: 20 minutes

Cook Time: 25 minutes

Total Time: 45 minutes

Nutrition Facts: (per serving):

Calories: 120

Fat: 3.1g

Salt: 121mg

Carbs: 23.4g

Fiber: 17.3gg

Sugar: 0.3g

Net Carbs: 6.1g

Protein: 6g

Cholesterol: 105mg

Potassium: 203mg

Vitamin D: 9mcg

Calcium: 80mg

Iron: 1mg

Ingredients:

1/4 cup coconut flour

2 tablespoons ground psyllium husks

4 egg whites

2 egg yolks

1 teaspoon paleo baking powder

1/2 tablespoon apple cider vinegar

1 cup water

1 teaspoon dried oregano (optional)

1 teaspoon dried thyme (optional)

Salt and pepper to taste

Instructions:

Preheat your oven to 350 degrees. Line a baking sheet with parchment paper.

With a hand mixer or whisk, beat the egg whites until they form a foam with stiff peaks. Set aside.

Mix all remaining ingredients in a separate bowl. Gently fold in the egg whites.

Form four thick, evenly sized rolls from your dough and place on the baking sheet. (Thickness is important so buns don't flatten.)

Bake for 40 minutes, or until cooked all the way through. If you cut one ope58.nd it still is moist, place them (even the one you have cut open) back in the oven for a few more minutes.

Remove from your oven and serve warm.

13. KT DR BISUITS

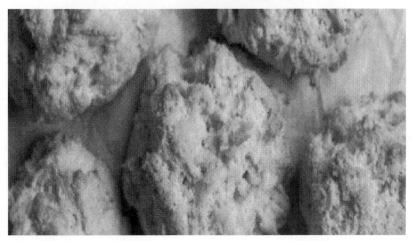

Prep Time : 10 mins

Cook Time : 15 mins

Total Time : 25 mins

Nutrition Facts:

Calories - 247 - Calories from Fat - 198

Fat 22g - 34%

Saturated Fat 4g - 25%

Cholesterol 12mg - 4%

Sodium 107mg - 5%

Potassium 113mg - 3%

Carbohydrates 8g - 3%

Fiber 4g - 17%

Sugar 1g - 1%

Protein 7g - 14%

Ingredients

1 egg

77 g sour cream or coconut cream + 2 tsp. apple cider vinegar, at room temp

2 tablespoons water

1 tablespoon apple cider vinegar

96 g almond flour

63 g golden flaxseed meal or psyllium husk, finely ground

21 g coconut flour

20 g whey protein isolate or more almond flour

3 1/2 teaspoons baking powder

1 teaspoon xanthan gum or 1 TBS. flaxseed meal

1/2 teaspoon kosher salt

112 g organic grass-fed butter or 7 TBS. ghee/coconut oil

Instructions

Preheat oven to 450°F/230°C. Line a baking tray with parchment paper or a baking mat.

Add eggs, sour (or coconut) cream, water and apple cider vinegar to a medium bowl and whisk for a minute or two until fully mixed. Set aside.

Add almond flour, flaxseed meal, coconut flour, whey protein, baking powder, xanthan gum (or more flax) and kosher salt to a food processor and pulse until very thoroughly combined.

Add in the butter and pulse a few times until pea-sized. Pour in the egg and cream mixture, pulsing until combined. The dough will be very shaggy.

Drop 6 rounds of dough onto the prepared baking tray. Brush with melted butter and bake for 15-20 minutes until deep golden. Allow to cool for 10 minutes before serving. These guys keep well, stored in an airtight container at room temperature, for 3-4 days.

You can freeze the shaped biscuit dough for 1-2 months, and bake straight from the freezer as needed.

14. RSMR KT BAGELS

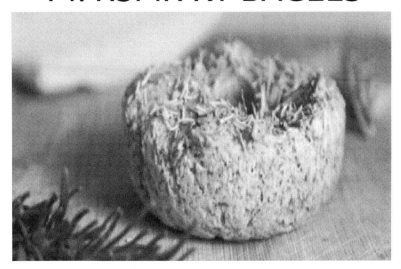

Cook Time: 55 minutes (10 minutes active)

Nutrition Facts: (Per Serving):

Calories: 285

Protein: 13g

Carbs: 12g

Fiber: 7.5g

Net Carbs: 4.5g

Sugar: 1.75g

Fat: 22.5g

Saturated Fat: 2g

Polyunsaturated: 0.25g

Monounsaturated: 0.5g

Trans fat: 0g

Cholesterol: 46mg

Sodium: 82.5mg

Potassium: 91mg

Vitamin A: 1mg

Vitamin C: 0mg

Calcium: 10mg

Iron: 10mg

Ingredients:

1 1/2 cups almond flour

3/4 teaspoon baking soda

3/4 teaspoon xanthan gum

1/4 teaspoon salt

3 tablespoons psyllium husk powder

1 whole egg

3 egg whites

1/2 cup warm water

1 tablespoon rosemary, chopped

Avocado oil

Instructions:

Preheat oven to 250F.

Mix almond flour, xanthan gum, baking soda and salt together in a bowl.

In a separate bowl, whisk eggs and warm water together. Stir in psyllium husk until there are no clumps.

Add liquid ingredients to dry ingredients.

Coat bagel mold with avocado oil.

Press dough into mold.

Sprinkle rosemary on top.

Place in oven and bake for 45 minutes.

Remove and cool for 15 minutes before slicing.

15. KETO TURMRI CULIFLWR BUNS

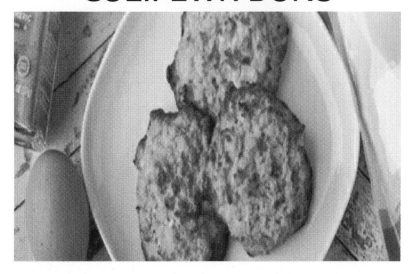

Prep Time: 30 mins

Cook Time: 30 mins

Nutrition Facts:

Total Fat - 2.1g

21% Cholesterol - 62mg

6% Sodium - 151.7mg

2% Total Carbohydrate 6.6g

Sugars - 2.4g

9% Protein - 4.5g

2% Vitamin A - 26.7µg

79% Vitamin C - 47.2mg

3% Calcium - 31.2mg

4% Magnesium - 17mg

Ingredients

1 medium head of cauliflower or about 2 cups of firmly packed cauliflower rice (see directions for making the cauliflower rice)

2 eggs

2 tablespoons coconut flour

¼ teaspoon ground turmeric

pinch each of salt and pepper

Instructions

Preheat oven to 400°F.

Line a baking sheet with parchment paper and set aside.

Take your cauliflower and use a sharp knife to cut off the base. Pull off any green parts and use your hands to break the cauliflower into florets. Give the florets a quick rinse and pat dry.

Next, make cauliflower rice by placing the florets into the bowl of a food processor with the "S" blade. Pulse for about 30 seconds until the cauliflower is about the size of rice. You should have about two cups of firmly packed cauliflower rice.

Place the cauliflower rice into a microwavable-safe bowl with about a teaspoon of water. Cover with plastic wrap and poke a few holes to let the steam escape. Microwave the cauliflower rice for about 3 minutes. Alternatively, you can steam the cauliflower rice on the stovetop in a steamer basket.

Uncover the bowl and let the cauliflower rice cool for about 5 minutes. Then, use a large spoon to put the cauliflower rice into a nut milk bag or a clean dish towel. Squeeze the excess moisture out, being careful not to burn your hands.

Pour the cauliflower rice into a medium mixing bowl and stir in the eggs, turmeric, and a pinch of salt and black pepper.

Use your hands to form the mixture into 6 buns, placing them on the baking sheet.

Bake for 25-30 minutes or until the top becomes slightly browned.

The cauliflower buns are best served hot right out of the oven. They do not refrigerate or re-heat well (they will get mushy), but they are so delicious that you'll no doubt eat them right away

16. LW CRB KETO ALMND FLUR BISUITS

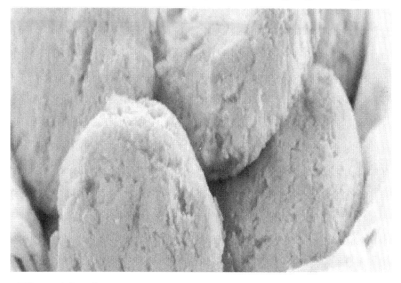

Prep Time 10 minutes

Cook Time 15 minutes

Total Time 25 minutes

Nutrition Facts:

Calories 164

Fat - 15g

Protein - 5g

Total Carbs - 4g

Net Carbs - 2g

Fiber - 2g

Sugar - 1g

Ingredients

2 cup Blanched almond flour

2 tsp Gluten-free baking powder

1/2 tsp Sea salt

2 large Egg (beaten)

1/3 cup Butter (measured solid, then melted; can use ghee or coconut oil for dairy-free)

Instructions

Preheat the oven to 350 degrees F (177 degrees C). Line a baking sheet with parchment paper.

Mix dry ingredients together in a large bowl. Stir in wet ingredients.

Scoop tablespoonfuls of the dough onto the lined baking sheet (a cookie scoop is the fastest way). Form into rounded biscuit shapes (flatten slightly with your fingers).

Bake for about 15 minutes, until firm and golden. Cool on the baking sheet.

17. Cranberry Jalapeño "Cornbread" Muffins

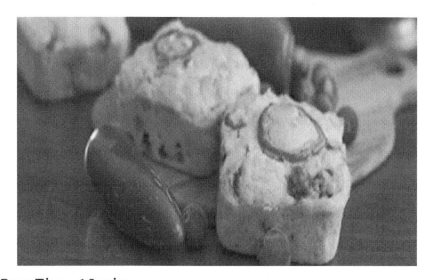

Prep Time : 10 mins

Cook Time: 30 mins

Total Time : 40 mins

Nutrition Facts:

Calories 157 - Calories from Fat - 101

Fat 11.22g - 17%

Saturated Fat 7.11g - 36%

Cholesterol 128mg - 43%

Sodium 362mg - 15%

Carbohydrates 7.08g - 2%

Fiber 3.84g - 15%

Protein 5.21g - 10%

Ingredients

- 1 cup coconut flour (I used Bob's Red Mill)
- 1/3 cup Swerve Sweetener or other erythritol
- 1 tbsp baking powder
- 1/2 tsp salt
- 7 large eggs, lightly beaten
- 1 cup unsweetened almond milk
- 1/2 cup butter, melted OR avocado oil
- 1/2 tsp vanilla
- 1 cup fresh cranberries, cut in half
- 3 tbsp minced jalapeño peppers
- 1 jalapeño, seeds removed, sliced into 12 slices, for garnish

Instructions

Preheat oven to 325F and grease a muffin tin well or line with paper liners.

In a medium bowl, whisk together coconut flour, sweetener, baking powder and salt. Break up any clumps with the back of a fork.

Stir in eggs, melted butter and almond milk and stir vigorously. Stir in vanilla extract and continue to stir until mixture is smooth and well combined. Stir in chopped cranberries and jalapeños.

Divide batter evenly among prepared muffin cups and place one slice of jalapeño on top of each.

Bake 25 to 30 minutes or until tops are set and a tester inserted in the center comes out clean. Let cool 10 minutes in pan, then transfer to a wire rack to cool completely.

18. KT BAGEL

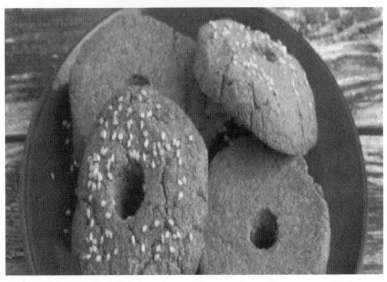

Prep Time 15 minutes

Cook Time 12 minutes

Total Time 27 minutes

Nutrition Facts:

Calories - 360

Fat - 28g

Protein - 21g

Total Carbs - 8g

Net Carbs - 5g

Fiber - 3g

Sugar - 1g

Ingredients

    1 cup (120 g) of almond flour

    1/4 cup (28 g) of coconut flour

    1 Tablespoon (7 g) of psyllium husk powder

    1 teaspoon (2 g) of baking powder

    1 teaspoon (3 g) of garlic powder

    pinch salt

    2 medium eggs (88 g)

    2 teaspoons (10 ml) of white wine vinegar

    2 1/2 Tablespoons (38 ml) of ghee, melted

    1 Tablespoon (15 ml) of olive oil

    1 teaspoon (5 g) of sesame seeds

Instructions

Preheat the oven to 320°F (160°C).

Combine the almond flour, coconut flour, psyllium husk powder, baking powder, garlic powder and salt in a bowl.

In a separate bowl, whisk the eggs and vinegar together. Slowly drizzle in the melted ghee (which should not be piping hot) and whisk in well.

Add the wet mixture to the dry mixture and use a wooden spoon to combine well. Leave to sit for 2-3 minutes.

Divide the mixture into 4 equal-sized portions. Using your hands, shape the mixture into a round shape and place onto a tray lined with parchment paper. Use a small spoon or apple corer to make the center hole.

Brush the tops with olive oil and scatter over the sesame seeds.

Bake in the oven for 20-25 minutes until cooked through. Allow to cool slightly before enjoying!

19. KETO BRKFST PIZZ

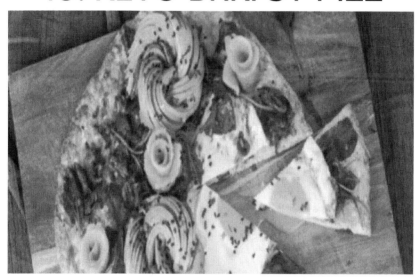

Prep Time:10 minutes

Cook Time :10 minutes

Total Time :20 minutes

Nutrition Facts:

Calories: 470

Total Fat: 37g

Saturated Fat: 15g

Trans Fat: 1g

Unsaturated Fat: 20g

Cholesterol: 248mg

Sodium: 840mg

Carbohydrates: 4g

Fiber: 1g

Sugar: 1g

Protein: 28g

Ingredients:

    2 cups grated cauliflower

    2 tablespoons coconut flour

    1/2 teaspoon salt

    4 eggs

    1 tablespoon psyllium husk powder (Use a mold-free brand like this one)

    Toppings: smoked Salmon, avocado, herbs, spinach, olive oil

Instructions:

Preheat the oven to 350 degrees. Line a pizza tray or sheet pan with parchment.

In a mixing bowl, add all ingredients except toppings and mix until combined. Set aside for 5 minutes to allow coconut flour and psyllium husk to absorb liquid and thicken up.

Carefully pour the breakfast pizza base onto the pan. Use your hands to mold it into a round, even pizza crust.

Bake for 15 minutes, or until golden brown and fully cooked.

Remove from the oven and top breakfast pizza with your chosen toppings. Serve warm.

20. CNUT FLUR
PIZZA CRUST

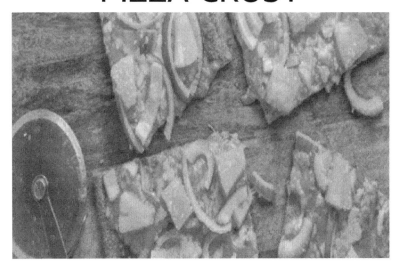

Prep Time: 10 mins

Cook Time: 20 mins

Total Time: 30 mins

Nutrition Facts:

Calories - 496 Calories from Fat - 297

Fat 33g - 51%

Saturated Fat 15g - 94%

Sodium 885mg - 38%

Carbohydrates 13g - 4%

Fiber 5g - 21%

Sugar 14g - 16%

Protein 35g - 70%

Ingredients

- 3/4 cup coconut flour clumps removed
- 3 tablespoons psyllium husk powder
- 1 teaspoon garlic powder
- 1/2 teaspoon Salt I love this Himalayan pink salt
- 1 teaspoon apple cider vinegar
- 1/2 teaspoon baking soda
- 3 eggs
- 1 cup boiling water

Instructions

Preheat oven to 350F.

Mix coconut flour with psyllium husk powder, garlic powder and salt until fully-incorporated.

Add in apple cider vinegar, baking soda and eggs. Mix together.

Mix boiling water in, and stir until incorporated. If the dough is too sticky, add in more coconut flour until it is the desired consistency. The dough will naturally be kind of sticky though, so you may want to use wet fingers to spread out the dough.

Spread dough out on a baking sheet to the desired thickness. I like mine to be pretty thin, so my dough usually covers the entire baking sheet.

Place in a preheated oven for 15-20 minutes, or until edges begin to brown.

Top with sauce, cheese and desired toppings and place back in the oven until the cheese is melted.

21. MINI PL PIZZ BSS CRUSTS

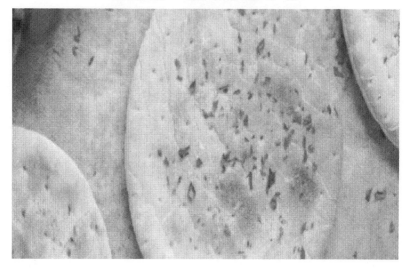

Prep Time: 10 min

Cook Time: 13 min

Ready In: 23 min

Nutrition Facts:

Calories: 125kcal

Carbohydrates: 6g

Protein: 8g

Fat: 1g

Fiber: 3g

Vitamin A: 1%

Vitamin C: 2%

Calcium: 1%

Iron: 2%

Ingredients

For the coconut flour option

8 large egg whites for thicker bases, use 5 whole eggs and 3 egg whites

1/4 cup coconut flour sifted

1/2 tsp baking powder

Spices of choice salt, pepper, Italian spices

Extra coconut flour to dust very lightly

For the almond flour option

8 large egg whites

1/2 cup almond flour

1/2 tsp baking powder

Spices of choice salt, pepper, Italian spices

For the pizza sauce

1/2 cup Mutti tomato sauce

2 cloves garlic crushed

1/4 tsp sea salt

1 tsp dried basil

Instructions

To make the pizza bases/crusts

In a large mixing bowl, whisk the eggs/egg whites until opaque. Sift in the coconut flour or almond flour and whisk very well until clumps are removed. Add the baking powder, mixed spices and continue to whisk until completely combined.

On low heat, heat up a small pan and grease lightly.Once frying pan is hot, pour the batter in the pan and ensure it is fully coated. Cover the pan with a lid/tray for 3-4 minutes or until bubbles start to appear on top. Flip, cook for an extra 2 minutes and remove from pan- Keep an eye on this, as it can burn out pretty quickly.

Continue until all the batter is used up.Allow pizza bases to cool. Once cool, use a skewer and poke holes roughly over the top, for even cooking. Dust very lightly with a dash of coconut flour.

To make the sauce

Combine all the ingredients together and let sit at room temperature for at least 30 minutes- This thickens up.

For a crispy pizza base, bake in the oven for 3-4 minutes prior to adding your toppings.If you want to freeze them, allow pizza bases to cool completely before topping with a dash of coconut flour and a thin layer of pizza sauce. Ensure each pizza base is divided with parchment paper before placing in the freezer.

22. KT ZUHINI BRD WITH WALNUT CRUST

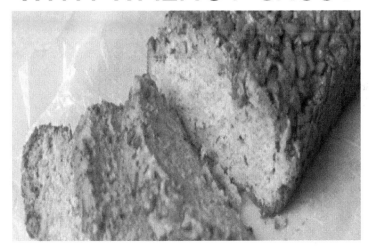

Prep Time: 10 minutes

Cook Time: 55 minutes

Total Time: 1 hour 5 minutes

Nutrition Facts:

Calories: 171

Total Fat: 15g

Carbohydrates: 5g

Fiber: 3g

Sugar: 2g

Protein: 5g

Ingredient

- 3 large eggs
- ½ cup olive oil
- 1 teaspoon vanilla extract
- 2 1/2 cups almond flour
- 1 1/2 cups erythritol
- ½ teaspoon salt
- 1 1/2 teaspoons baking powder
- ½ teaspoon nutmeg
- 1 teaspoon ground cinnamon
- ¼ teaspoon ground ginger
- 1 cup grated zucchini
- ½ cup chopped walnuts

Instruction

Preheat oven to 350°F. Whisk together the eggs, oil, and vanilla extract. Set to the side.

In another bowl, mix together the almond flour, erythritol, salt, baking powder, nutmeg, cinnamon, and ginger. Set to the side.

Using a cheesecloth or paper towel, take the zucchini and squeeze out the excess water.

Then, whisk the zucchini into the bowl with the eggs.

Slowly add the dry ingredients into the egg mixture using a hand mixer until fully blended.

Lightly spray a 9x5 loaf pan, and spoon in the zucchini bread mixture.

Then, spoon in the chopped walnuts on top of the zucchini bread. Press walnuts into the batter using a spatula.

Bake for 60-70 minutes at 350°F or until the walnuts on top look browned.

23. KETO PUMPKIN BRD

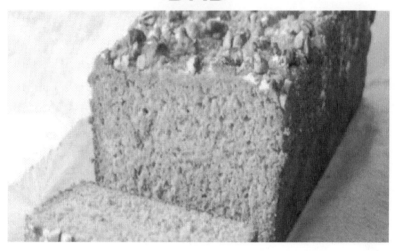

Prep Time : 10 minutes

Cook Time: 50 minutes

Total Time: 1 hour

Nutrition Facts:

Calories - 215

Fat - 18g

Protein - 8g

Total Carbs - 9g

Net Carbs - 4g

Fiber - 5g

Sugar - 2g

Ingredients

1/2 cup butter, softened

2/3 cup erythritol sweetener, like Swerve

4 eggs large

3/4 cup pumpkin puree, canned (see notes for fresh)

1 tsp vanilla extract

1 1/2 cup almond flour

1/2 cup coconut flour

4 tsp baking powder

1 tsp cinnamon

1/2 tsp nutmeg

1/4 tsp ginger

1/8 tsp cloves

1/2 tsp salt

Instructions

Preheat the oven to 350°F. Grease a 9"x5" loaf pan, and line with parchment paper.

In a large mixing bowl, cream the butter and sweetener together until light and fluffy.

Add the eggs, one at a time, and mix well to combine.

Add the pumpkin puree and vanilla, and mix well to combine.

In a separate bowl, stir together the almond flour, coconut flour, baking powder, cinnamon, nutmeg, ginger, cloves, salt. Break up any lumps of almond flour or coconut flour.

Add the dry ingredients to the wet ingredients, and stir to combine. (Optionally, add up to 1/2 cup of mix-ins, like chopped nuts or chocolate chips.)

Pour the batter into the prepared loaf pan. Bake for 45 - 55 minutes, or until a toothpick inserted into the center of the loaf comes out clean.

If the bread is browning too quickly, you can cover the pan with a piece of aluminum foil.

24. LOW CRB BLUBRR ENGLISH MUFFIN BRD LOAF

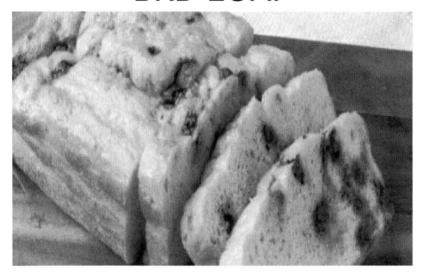

Prep Time: 15 minutes

Cook Time: 45 minutes

Total Time: 1 hour

Nutrition Facts:

Calories 156 - Calories from Fat - 117

Fat 13g - 20%

Doc Julian

Saturated Fat 3g - 19%

Cholesterol 78mg - 26%

Sodium 171mg - 7%

Potassium 192mg - 5%

Carbohydrates 4g - 1%

Fiber 1g - 4%

Sugar 1g - 1%

Protein 5g - 10%

Vitamin A 215IU - 4%

Vitamin C 0.6mg - 1%

Calcium 106mg - 11%

Iron 1mg - 6%

Ingredients

   1/2 cup almond butter or cashew or peanut butter

   1/4 cup butter ghee or coconut oil

   1/2 cup almond flour

   1/2 tsp salt

   2 tsp baking powder

   1/2 cup almond milk unsweetened

   5 eggs beaten

   1/2 cup blueberries

Instructions

Preheat oven to 350 degrees F.

In a microwavable bowl melt nut butter and butter together for

30 seconds, stir until combined well.

In a large bowl, whisk almond flour, salt and baking powder together. Pour the nut butter mixture into the large bowl and stir to combine.

Whisk the almond milk and eggs together then pour into the bowl and stir well.

Drop in fresh blueberries or break apart frozen blueberries and gently stir into the batter.

Line a loaf pan with parchment paper and lightly grease the parchment paper as well.

Pour the batter into the loaf pan and bake 45 minutes or until a toothpick in center comes out clean.

Cool for about 30 minutes then remove from pan.

Slice and toast each slice before serving.

25. CINNMN ALMND FLUR BRD

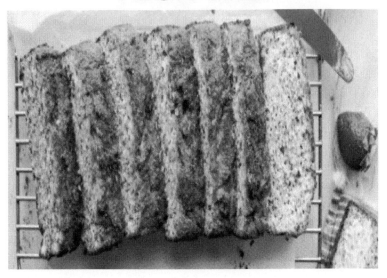

Prep Time: 10 minutes

Cook Time: 30 minutes

Total Time: 40 minutes

Nutrition Facts:

Calories: 208

Total Fat: 18g

Saturated Fat: 5g

Trans Fat: 0g

Unsaturated Fat: 12g

Cholesterol: 70mg

Sodium: 238mg

Carbohydrates: 7g

Fiber: 4g

Sugar: 1g

Protein: 7g

Ingredients

2 cups fine blanched almond flour
(I use Bob's Red Mill)

2 tbsp coconut flour

1/2 tsp sea salt

1 tsp baking soda

1/4 cup Flax seed meal or chia meal

5 Eggs and 1 egg white whisked

together

1.5 tsp Apple cider vinegar or lemon juice

2 tbsp maple syrup or honey

2–3 tbsp of clarified butter (melted) or Coconut oil; divided.

Vegan butter also works

1 tbsp cinnamon plus extra for topping

Optional chia seed to sprinkle of top before baking

Instructions

Preheat oven to 350F. Line an 8×4 bread pan with parchment

paper at the bottom and grease the sides.

In a large bowl, mix together your almond flour, coconut flour, salt, baking soda, flaxseed meal or chia meal, and 1/2 tablespoon of cinnamon.

In another small bowl, whisk together your eggs and egg white. Then add in your maple syrup (or honey), apple cider vinegar, and melted butter (1.5 to 2 tbsp).

Mix wet ingredients into dry. Be sure to remove any clumps that might have occurred from the almond flour or coconut flour.

Pour batter into a your greased loaf pan.

Bake at 350º for 30-35 minutes, until a toothpick inserted into center of loaf comes out clean.

Remove from and oven.Next, whisk together the other 1 to 2 tbsp of melted butter (or oil) and mix it with 1/2 tbsp of cinnamon. Brush this on top of your cinnamon almond flour bread.

Cool and serve or store for later.

26. KET CHLT ZUCCHINI BREAD

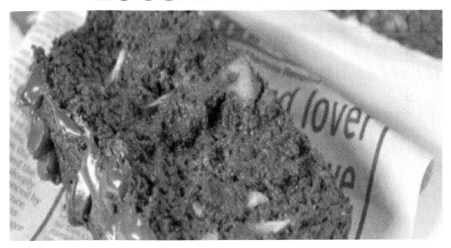

Prep Time: 10 mins

Cook Time: 50 mins

Total Time: 1 hr

Nutrition Facts:

Calories 185 - Calories from Fat - 154

Fat 17.1g - 26%

Carbohydrates 6.1g - 2%

Fiber 2.7g - 11%

Sugar 1.2g - 1%

Protein 4.9g - 10%

Doc Julian

Ingredients

Dry ingredients

1 1/2 cup almond flour (170g)

1/4 cup unsweetened cocoa powder (25g)

1 1/2 teaspoon baking soda

2 teaspoons ground cinnamon

1/4 teaspoon sea salt

1/2 cup sugar free crystal sweetener (Monk fruit or erythritol) (100g) or coconut sugar if refined sugar free

Wet ingredients

1 cup zucchini, finely grated measure packed, discard juice/liquid if there is some - about 2 small zucchini

1 large egg

1/4 cup + 2 tablespoon canned coconut cream 100ml

1/4 cup extra virgin coconut oil , melted, 60ml

1 teaspoon vanilla extract

1 teaspoon apple cider vinegar

Filling - optional

1/2 cup sugar free chocolate chips

1/2 cup chopped walnuts or nuts you like

Instructions

Preheat oven to 180C (375F). Line a baking loaf pan (9 inches x 5 inches) with parchment paper. Set aside.

Remove both extremity of the zucchinis, keep skin on.

Finely grate the zucchini using a vegetable grater. Measure the amount needed in a measurement cup. Make sure you press/pack them firmly for a precise measure and to squeeze out any liquid from the grated zucchini, I usually don't have any!. If you do, discard the liquid or keep for another recipe.

In a large mixing bowl, stir all the dry ingredients together: almond flour, unsweetened cocoa powder, sugar free crystal sweetener, cinnamon, sea salt and baking soda. Set aside.

Add all the wet ingredients into the dry ingredients : grated zucchini, coconut oil, coconut cream, vanilla, egg, apple cider vinegar.

Stir to combine all the ingredients together.

Stir in the chopped nuts and sugar free chocolate chips.

Transfer the chocolate bread batter into the prepared loaf pan.

Bake 50 - 55 minutes, you may want to cover the bread loaf with a piece of foil after 40 minute to avoid the top to darken too much, up to you.

The bread will stay slightly moist in the middle and firm up after fully cool down.

Cool down

Cool down 10 minutes in the loaf pan, then cool down on a cooling rack until it reach room temperature. It can take 4 hours as it is a thick bread. Don' slice the bread before it reach room temperature. If too hot in the center, it will be too oft and fall apart when you slice.

For a faster result, cool down 40 minutes at room temperature then pop in the fridge for 1 hour. The fridge will create an extra fudgy texture and the bread will be even easier to slice as it firms up.

Store in the fridge up to 4 days in a cake bow or airtight container.

27. LOW CARB GLUTN FR CRANBERRY BREAD

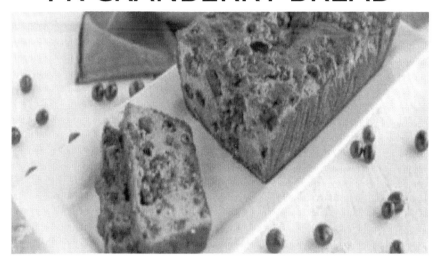

Prep Time: 10 minutes

Cook Time: 1 hour 15 minutes

Total Time: 1 hour 25 minutes

Nutrition Facts:

Calories 179 - Calories from Fat - 135

Fat 15g - 23%

Saturated Fat 4g - 25%

Cholesterol 72mg - 24%

Sodium 276mg - 12%

Potassium 38mg - 1%

Carbohydrates 7g - 2%

Fiber 2g - 8%

Sugar 1g - 1%

Protein 6.4g - 13%

Vitamin A 250IU - 5%

Calcium 80mg - 8%

Iron 1.1mg - 6%

    Net Carbs 5g

    % Carbs: 11.1%

    % Protein: 14.2%

    % Fat: 74.8%

Ingredients

2 cups almond flour

1/2 cup powdered erythritol or Swerve, see Note

1/2 teaspoon Steviva stevia powder see Note

1 1/2 teaspoons baking powder

1/2 teaspoon baking soda

1 teaspoon salt

4 tablespoons unsalted butter melted (or coconut oil)

1 teaspoon blackstrap molasses optional (for brown sugar flavor)

4 large eggs at room temperature

1/2 cup coconut milk

1 bag cranberries 12 ounces

Instructions

Preheat oven to 350 degrees; grease a 9-by-5 inch loaf pan and set aside.

In a large bowl, whisk together flour, erythritol, stevia, baking powder, baking soda, and salt; set aside.

In a medium bowl, combine butter, molasses, eggs, and coconut milk.

Mix dry mixture into wet mixture until well combined.

Fold in cranberries. Pour batter into prepared pan.

Bake until a toothpick inserted in the center of the loaf comes clean, about 1 hour and 15 minutes.

Transfer pan to a wire rack; let bread cool 15 minutes before removing from pan.

28. CNUT FLUR PSLLIUM HUSK BREAD

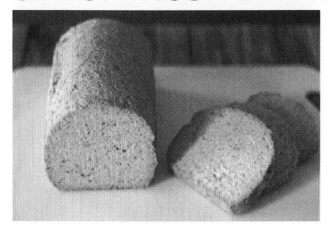

Prep Time 5 minutes

Cook Time 55 minutes

Total Time 1 hour

Nutrition Facts:

Calories 127 - Calories from Fat = 120

Fat 13.3g - 20%

Sodium 243mg - 11%

Carbohydrates 6g - 2%

Fiber 4.1g - 17%

Protein 3g - 6%

   Net Carbs 1.9g

   % Carbs: 5.5%

   % Protein: 8.6%

   % Fat: 85.9%

Ingredients

6 tablespoons whole psyllium husks 27g, may want to finely grind

3/4 cup warm water

1 cup coconut flour 125g

1 1/2 teaspoons baking soda

3/4 teaspoon sea salt

1 pint egg whites 2 cups (or use 8 whole eggs)

2 large eggs see note

1/2 cup olive oil

1/4 cup coconut oil melted

Instructions

Preheat oven to 350°F.

If not using silicone pan, grease or line pan with parchment paper. I used an 8x4-in pan.

Dump all ingredients into a food processor and pulse until well combined. If you don't have a food processor, you can use a mixing bowl with electric mixer.

Spread batter into 8x4 loaf pan. Smooth top.

Bake for 45-55 minutes or until edges are brown and toothpick inserted comes out clean.

Let bread sit in pan for 15 minutes. Remove bread from pan and allow to cool completely on rack.

29. CHEESY KT GRLI BREAD - USING MOZZARELLA DOUGH

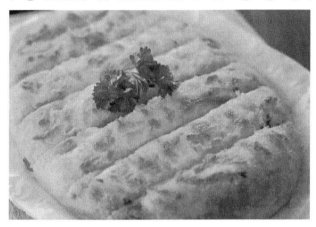

Prep Time: 10 mins

Cook Time: 15 mins

Total Time: 25 mins

Nutrition Facts:

Calories - 117.4 Calories from Fat - 88

Fat 9.8g - 15%

Carbohydrates 2.4g - 1%

Fiber 0.9g - 4%

Sugar 0.6g - 1%

Protein 6.2g - 12%

Ingredients

170 g pre shredded/grated cheese mozzarella

85 g almond meal/flour *see recipe notes below

2 tbsp cream cheese full fat

1 tbsp garlic crushed

1 tbsp parsley fresh or dried

1 tsp baking powder

pinch salt to taste

1 egg medium

Instructions

Place all the ingredients apart from the egg, in a microwaveable bowl. Stir gently to mix together. Microwave on HIGH for 1 minute.

Stir then microwave on HIGH for a further 30 seconds.

Add the egg then mix gently to make a cheesy dough.

Place on a baking tray and form into a garlic bread shape. Cut slices into the low-carb garlic bread.

Optional: Mix 2 tbsp melted butter, 1 tsp parsley and 1 tsp garlic. Brush over the top of the low-carb garlic bread, sprinkle with more cheese.

Bake at 220C/425F for 15 minutes, or until golden brown.

30. NUT-FR KETO BRD

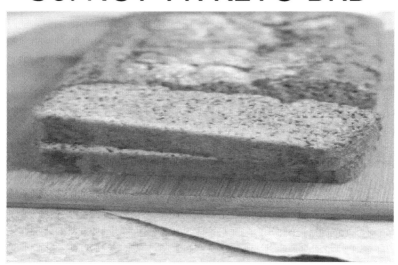

Prep Time: 15 minutes

Cook Time: 35 minutes

Total Time: 50 minutes

Nutrition Facts:

Calories 171 - Calories from Fat - 108

Fat 12g - 18%

Saturated Fat 2g - 13%

Cholesterol 62mg - 21%

Sodium 321mg - 14%

Potassium 91mg - 3%

Carbohydrates 8g - 3%

Fiber 6g - 25%

Protein 7g - 14%

Vitamin A 135IU - 3%

Calcium 60mg - 6%

Iron 2.2mg - 12%

Ingredients

9 eggs

2/3 cup coconut oil, softened yet not melted

2/3 cup coconut flour

2 tsp cream of tartar

1 tsp baking soda

3/4 tsp xanthan gum

1/4 tsp salt

Optional

1 tsp sesame seeds

Instructions

Preheat oven to 350 degrees and grease 9×5 bread loaf pan (* see note below).

To a mixing bowl, add eggs and, using an electric mixer, mix on high for 2 minutes. Add coconut oil and mix on high until well-incorporated with eggs.

To a separate bowl, add dry ingredients and whisk together. With electric mixer turned to low, slowly add dry ingredients to wet ingredients and mix until fully incorporated and dough is formed. Pour dough into prepared loaf pan, top with sesame seeds, and bake for 35 minutes.

Remove pan from oven, carefully flip pan upside down on to cutting board or plate to remove bread from pan, and allow bread to cool completely before cutting into slices.

31. KETO CNUT FLUR FLATBREAD

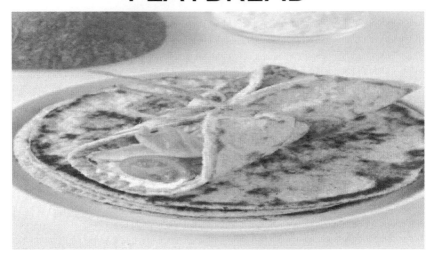

Prep Time: 10 mins

Cook Time: 5 mins

Total Time: 15 mins

Nutrition Facts:

Calories 66 - Calories from Fat - 30

Fat 3.3g - 5%

Carbohydrates 7.3g - 2%

Fiber 4.7g - 20%

Sugar 2g - 2%

Protein 2g - 4%

Ingredients

2 tablespoons psyllium husk (9g)

1/2 cup coconut flour fine, fresh, no lumps (60g)

1 cup lukewarm water (240ml)

1 tablespoon olive oil (15ml)

1/4 teaspoons baking soda

1/4 teaspoons salt - optional

Cooking

1 teaspoon olive oil to rub/oil the non stick pan

Instructions

Make the dough

In a medium mixing bowl, combine the psyllium husk and coconut flour (if lumps are in your flour use a fork to smash them BEFORE measuring the flour, amount must be precise).

Add in the lukewarm water (I used tap water about 40C/bath temperature), olive oil, and baking soda. Give a good stir with a spatula, then use your hands to knead the dough. Add salt now if you want. I never add the salt in contact with baking soda to avoid deactivating the leaving agent.

Knead for 1 minute. The dough is moist and it gets softer and slightly dryer as you go. It should come together easily to form a dough as on my picture. If not, too sticky, add more husk, 1/2 teaspoon at a time, knead for 30 sec and see how it goes. The dough will always be a bit moist but it shouldn't stick to your hands at all. It must come together as a dough.

Set aside 10 minute in the mixing bowl.

Now the dough must be soft, elastic and hold well together, it is ready to roll.

Roll/ shape the flatbread

Cut the dough into 4 even pieces, roll each pieces into a small ball.

Place one of the dough ball between two pieces of parchment paper, press the ball with your hand palm to stick it well to the paper and start rolling with a rolling pin as thin as you like a bread. My breads are 20 cm diameter (8 inches) and I made 6 flatbread with this recipe.

Un peel the first layer of parchment paper from your flatbread. Use a lid to cut out round flatbread. Keep the outside dough to reform a ball and roll more flatbread - that is how I make 2 extra flatbread from the 4 balls above! Cook in non stick pan

Warm a non stick tefal crepe/ pancake pan under medium/ high heat- or use any non stick pan of your choice, the one you would use for your pancakes.

Add one teaspoon of olive oil or vegetable oil of your choice onto a piece of absorbent paper. Rub the surface of the pan to make sure it is slightly oiled. Don't leave any drops of oil or the bread will fry!

Flip over the flatbread on the hot pan and peel off carefully the last piece of parchment paper.

Cook for 2-3 minutes on the first side, flip over using a spatula and cook for 1-2 more minute on the other side.

Cool down the flatbread on a plate and use as a sandwich wrap later or enjoy hot as a side dish. I recommend a drizzle of olive oil, crushed garlic and herbs before serving! (optional but delish!)

Repeat the rolling, cooking for the next 3 flatbread. Make sure you rub the oiled absorbent paper onto the saucepan each time to avoid the bread to stick to the pan.

Store in the pantry in an airtight box or on a plate covered with plastic wrap to keep them soft, for up to 3 days.

Rewarm in the same pan or if you want to give them a little crisp rewarm in the hot oven on a baking sheet for 1-2 minutes at 150C.

32. HOMEMADE NUT ND SD KETO BRD

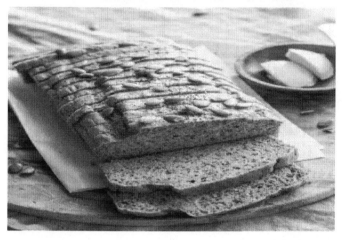

Prep Time : 20 mins

Cook Time : 1 hr

Total Time : 1 hr 20 mins

Nutrition Facts:

Calories: 191kcal

Carbohydrates: 6g

Protein: 5g

Fat: 16g

Saturated Fat: 1g

Fiber: 3g

Ingredients

1 1/4 cup almond flour

5 eggs (6 if you want extra fluffy)

1/3 cup coconut oil or avocado oil

1 tsp white vinegar or apple cider vinegar

1/2 tsp sea salt

dash of black pepper

Optional 1 tsp spice mix of choice (garlic, rosemary, Italian, etc.).

1 – 2 tsp poppyseed (plus extra for topping)

3 to 4 tbsp tapioca flour (if you are using more egg, add 4 tbsp).

1/2 tsp baking soda

1/4 cup chia meal (just grind chia seed in a coffee grinder or blender) or use ground flaxseed

Pumpkin seed for topping and Extra poppyseed

Instructions

Preheat oven to 350. Grease a 9×5 bread pan or line with parchment paper. Set aside. For higher rising bread, use an 8×4 pan.

In a small bowl, whisk your eggs, oil, and vinegar.

In another bowl, combine your flours, poppyseed, and seasonings.

Add your wet ingredients to dry ingredients and mix thoroughly.

Pour batter into greased pan and top with additional

pumpkin seeds and and additional poppyseed.

Bake covered for 20 minutes. Then uncover and continue to bake for additional 15-20 more or golden and knife in the centre comes out clean.

Should be around 35-45 minutes all together depending on your oven. If you used 8×4 or are baking at higher elevation, you might need to bake longer.

Remove from oven and let cool.

Wrap the paleo bread in foil or plastic wrap, slice and store in container. Keeps well in fridge for up to 7 days or freezer for up to 3 months.

33. CINNMN & HN KT BREAD

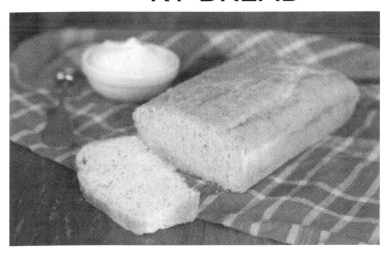

Prep Time: 15 minutes

Cooking Time: 30 minutes

Total Time: 45 minutes

Nutrition Facts:

Calories 319 - Calories from Fat - 261

Fat 29g - 45%

Saturated Fat 10g - 50%

Cholesterol 93mg - 31%

Sodium 531mg - 22%

Doc Julian

Potassium 91mg - 3%

Carbohydrates 8g - 3%

Fiber 4g - 16%

Sugar 1g - 1%

Protein 8g - 16%

Vitamin A 545IU - 11%

Calcium 108mg - 11%

Iron 1.6mg - 9%

Ingredients

Primal

   1 ½ cups blanched almond flour (165 g)

   4 large eggs, separated

   1 tablespoon egg white protein powder (5 g)

   5 tablespoons unsalted butter, melted (70 g)

   ¼ teaspoon kosher salt (1.2 ml)

   3 teaspoons aluminum-free baking powder (15 ml)

   1 ½ teaspoons cinnamon (7 ml)

   1 tablespoon honey (15 ml)

   ¼ teaspoon cream of tartar (1.2 ml)

   Garlic, Dill & Cheddar Keto Bread

Ingredients

   1 ½ cups blanched almond flour (165 g)

   4 large eggs, separated

   1 tablespoon egg white protein powder (5 g)

   5 tablespoons unsalted butter, melted and cooled (70 g)

¼ teaspoon kosher salt (1.2 ml)

3 teaspoons aluminum-free baking powder (15 ml)

¼ teaspoon cream of tartar (1.2 ml)

1 teaspoon garlic powder (5 ml)

1 teaspoon dried dill (5 ml)

1 cup grated cheddar cheese (90g)

Instructions

Primal

Preheat oven to 375º F/190º C.

Lightly grease an 8.5 x 4.5 loaf pan. For easiest release, cover the bottom of the loaf pan with lightly greased parchment paper.

In a food processor, combine the almond flour, egg yolks, egg white protein powder, butter, salt and baking powder.

*If making cinnamon & honey bread, add the cinnamon and honey.

*If making garlic, dill & cheddar bread, add the garlic powder, dill and cheddar.

Process just until the ingredients come together into a ball of dough.

In the bowl of an electric mixer, combine the egg whites and cream of tartar. Using the whisk attachment, whisk until the egg whites are big and fluffy and soft peaks form (when the whisk is lifted out of the egg whites, a soft peak should form, then fall slightly).

Pour 1/3 of the egg whites into the food processor. Pulse until combined, scraping down the sides as needed. Add another 1/3 of the egg whites, and pulse again until combined into a wet batter.

Primal

Scrape the dough out of the food processor into the bowl with the remaining egg whites. Use a spatula to gently fold the egg whites into the dough. Gently fold and mix until there are no white streaks, but be gentle; the air in the egg whites helps the dough rise into a loaf with a light texture.

Scrape the batter into the loaf pan. Bake 30 minutes.

Let cool for at least 30 minutes before removing from the loaf pan. Try to let the loaf cool completely on a wire rack before slicing.

Primal keto bread keeps for 1 to 2 days on the counter with simply a light towel over the top of it. For longer storage (3 to 5 days), keep the keto bread wrapped lightly in a towel inside a sealed plastic bag in the refrigerator.

34. CHS SKILLT BREAD

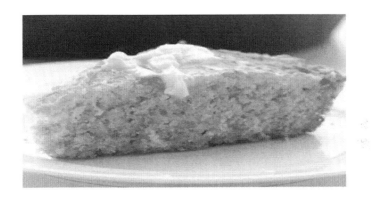

Prep Time : 10 mins

Cook Time : 16 mins

Total Time : 26 mins

Nutrition Facts:

Calories 357 Calories from Fat - 276

Fat 30.63g - 47%

Carbohydrates 7.9g - 3%

Fiber 4.77g - 19%

Protein 12.48g - 25%

Ingredients

1 tbsp butter for the skillet

2 cups almond flour

1/2 cup flax seed meal

2 tsp baking powder

1/2 tsp salt

1 & 1/2 cups shredded Cheddar cheese divided

3 large eggs lightly beaen

1/2 cup butter melted

3/4 cup almond milk

Instructions

Preheat oven to 425F. Add 1 tbsp butter to a 10-inch oven-proof skillet and place in oven.

In a large bowl, whisk together almond flour, flax seed meal, baking powder, salt and 1 cup of the shredded cheddar cheese.

Stir in the eggs, melted butter and almond milk until thoroughly combined.

Remove hot skillet from oven (remember to put on your oven mitts), and swirl butter to coat sides.

Pour batter into pan and smooth the top. Sprinkle with remaining 1/2 cup cheddar.

Bake 16 to 20 minutes, or until browned around the edges and set through the middle. Cheese on top should be nicely browned.

Remove and let cool 15 minutes.

35. KETO LW CARB BNN BRD

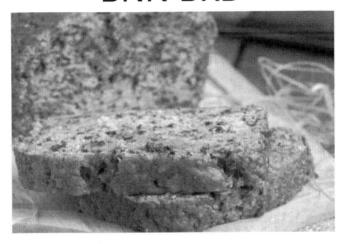

Prep Time: 10 minutes

Cook Time: 1 hour

Total Time: 1 hour 10 minutes

Nutrition Facts:

Calories - 224

Fat - 20g

Protein - 8g

Total Carbs - 6g

Net Carbs - 2g

Fiber - 4g

Sugar - 1g

Ingredients

3 overripe banana, mashed

3 large eggs

2 cups almond flour

1/4 cup olive oil or coconut oil

1 tsp baking soda

stevia or preferred sweetener (add as much as desired depending on your level of sweetness)

1/2 cup walnuts (optional)

coconut oil for spraying/greasing the pan

Instructions

Preheat oven at 350F.

In a food processor or a bowl, add eggs and beat. Add mashed banana. Add olive oil. Mix.

In a separate bowl mix together the almond flour, baking soda, and stevia.

Combine the two mixtures together until well blended. Toss in the walnuts.

Spray/grease the loaf pan with coconut oil and pour batter.

Bake for 60 minutes. Use a tester or a toothpick, if it comes out clean then it's cooked!

36. KT FTHD ROLLS

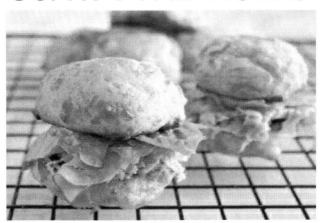

Prep Time : 10 minutes

Cook Time : 15 minutes

Total Time : 25 minutes

Nutrition Facts:

Calories 216 Calories from Fat - 144

Fat 16g - 25%

Saturated Fat 4g - 25%

Cholesterol 82mg - 27%

Sodium 183mg - 8%

Potassium 277mg - 8%

Carbohydrates 6g - 2%

Fiber 2g - 8%

Sugar 1g - 1%

Protein 11g - 22%

Vitamin A 285IU - 6%

Calcium 319mg - 32%

Iron 1.3mg - 7%

Net Carbs 4g - 8%

Ingredients

  2 oz cream cheese

  3/4 cup shredded mozzarella

  1 egg beaten

  1/4 tsp garlic powder

  1/3 cup almond flour

  2 tsp baking powder

  1/2 cup shredded cheddar cheese

Instructions

  Preheat the oven to 425°

In a small bowl, add cream cheese and mozzarella. Microwave on high for 20 seconds at a time until melted.

In a separate bowl, whisk egg until beaten. Add dry ingredients and mix well.

Work mozzarella/cc mixture into dough. Dough will be sticky. Stir in cheddar cheese.

Spoon dough onto plastic wrap. Dust the top of it with almond flour.

Fold the plastic wrap over the dough and gently start working into a ball.

Cover and refrigerate 30 minutes.

Cut dough ball into 4. Roll each section into a ball. Cut the ball in half. This is your top and bottom bun!

Sit cut side down on parchment paper or very well greased sheet pan.

Bake 10-12 minutes or until golden and set up.

37. KETO CINNAMON CLUD BREAD

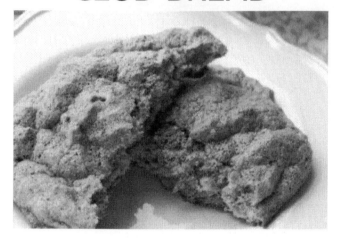

Prep Time: 10 minutes

Cook Time: 25 minutes

Total Time: 35 minutes

Nutrition Facts:

Calories: 199kcal

Carbohydrates: 10g

Protein: 3g

Fat: 19g Saturated Fat: 11g

Polyunsaturated Fat: 0g

Monounsaturated Fat: 0g

Trans Fat: 0g

Cholesterol: 118mg

Sodium: 167mg

Potassium: 67mg

Fiber: 0g

Sugar: 1g

Vitamin A: 15.1%

Vitamin C: 0%

Calcium: 4.7%

Iron: 2.4%

Ingredients:

    1/4 cup xylitol

    4 large eggs

    1/2 tsp baking powder

    1 tsp vanilla

    2 Tbsp sour cream

    1 Tbsp ground cinnamon

Instructions:

Preheat oven to 350 degrees F (176 C)

Place xylitol in a small mixing bowl. Using an egg separator over the bowl for your stand mixer, separate your eggs so that the egg whites go into the mixer bowl. Add the yolks to the bowl with the xylitol.

To the bowl with the egg yolks and xylitol, add vanilla, sour cream and cinnamon, mixing well after each addition. Set aside.

To the mixing bowl with the egg whites, add baking powder and beat on high speed for 5-7 minutes or until egg white mixture forms stiff peaks and holds it shape.

Fold the yolk mixture into the egg white mixture until just incorporated.

Make six mounds on a cookie sheet prepped with either parchment paper or a silpat style baking mat. Use the back of your spoon or spatula to smooth out the tops of the mounds to make them flat.

Bake at 350 degrees F (176 C) for 20 minutes or until the tops are just beginning to brown and the bread is set. Allow to cool before serving.

38. KT BRD ROLLS

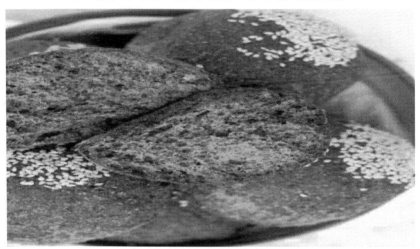

Prep Time: 15 minutes

Cook Time: 1 hour

Total Time: 1 hour, 15 minutes

Nutrition Facts:

Total Fat 14.6g - 22%

Total Carbohydrate 23.6g - 8%

Dietary Fiber 20.3g - 81%

Protein 6.5g- 13%

Ingredients

Flax Egg

3 tbsp ground flax seeds

1/2 cup + 1 tbsp water

Bread Roll Dough

1 1/4 cup almond flour

1/3 cup ground flax seeds

1/2 cup psyllium husk powder

1 tsp salt

2 1/2 tsp baking soda

1 1/4 tsp cream of tartar

1 1/4 cup water

Optional

2 tsp sesame seeds

Instructions

Preheat oven to 375 degrees and line baking sheet with parchment paper.

For the flax egg, to a small bowl, add flax seeds and water and whisk together. Allow to soak for 5 minutes.

In a medium bowl, add dry ingredients and whisk together until fully incorporated. Add flax egg and mix with electric mixer until well-combined.

In a small pot, bring water to boil.

With the electric mixer turned on, slowly pour boiling water over dough mixture. Mix until all ingredients are combined. Let dough rest for 5 minutes.

Form dough into 6 equal rolls (*see note below).

(Optional) To a shallow dish, add a small amount of water. To another shallow dish, add sesame seeds. Dip rolls one-by-one in water then sesame seeds to coat the top.

Place rolls on prepared baking dish and bake for 50 minutes. Turn oven off and crack oven door. Allow rolls to sit inside cooling oven for 10 additional minutes. Remove rolls from oven and allow to fully cool before serving.

39. ES OSI FLTBRD

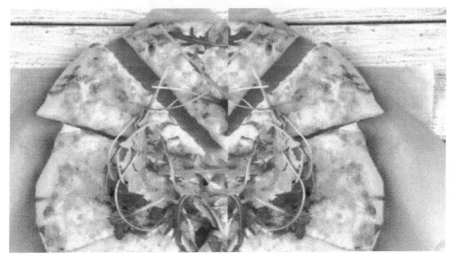

Nutrition Facts:

Calories; 36g

Fat (77.8% calories from fat);

22g Protein;

2g Carbohydrate;

0 Dietary Fiber.

Ingredients

3 eggs, room temp, separate out yolks

1/4 tsp cream of tartar

3 oz neufchatel cheese, cold (sub cottage cheese or ricotta)

stevia (or equiv), to taste

favorite herbs and spices, to taste

2 oz cheddar cheese (or Parmesan) shredded

Directions

Preheat oven to 300 F. Separate eggs. Beat egg whites with cream of tartar until stiff.

In a separate bowl, mix together egg yolks, spices/herbs of choice and cream cheese. Gently fold the yolk mix into the egg whites. Be careful not to break down the whites!

Scoop (don't pour) the batter into a circular pile on a lightly greased oven tray. Pile the batter as high as possible. (We're not going for Mt. Everest, though.)

Make the batter pile the size of your flatbread (usually 6 to 10 inches in diameter). Or, make 6 small piles – perfect for low carb buns.

Bake at 300 F in the oven for about 30 minutes.

Remove from oven and allow to cool on a rack. Your flatbread deflates a bit during this time, and becomes firmer.

Store your Oopsie flatbread in a loose-lid container on the counter, in the fridge or freezer (thaw before use).

When you are ready to use:

Slather or spray lightly with olive oil (or melted butter), top with grated cheddar or Parmesan (or desired cheese), and dark greens like spinach or arugula (both have 0.4g net carbs per cup).

Toast or broil in the oven until cheese is melted, bubbly and Oopsie flatbread is slightly browned. Toast longer at a lower temp for an extra crispy, crunchy flatbread.

40. KT PUMKIN CHI MUFFINS

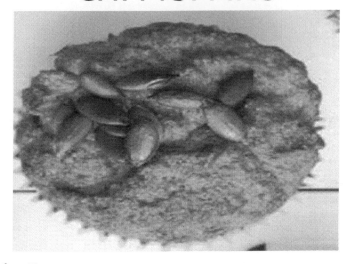

Nutrition Facts:

Calories from carbs - 6%,

protein - 14%,

fat - 80%

Total carbs - 6 grams

Fiber - 3.1 grams

Sugars - 1.4 grams

Saturated fat - 6.3 grams

Sodium - 188 mg

Magnesium - 54 mg

Potassium - 178 mg

Ingredients (makes 12 muffins)

Dry ingredients:

1 1/2 cups almond flour (150 g/ 5.3 oz)

1/4 cup ground chia seeds (32 g/ 1.1 oz)

1 tbsp gluten-free baking powder (you can make your own)

1 tbsp pumpkin pie spice mix (you can make your own)

1/4 cup Erythritol or Swerve, powdered (40 g / 1.4 oz) or other healthy low-carb sweetener from this list

Topping: 6 tbsp pumpkin seeds (pepitas) (25 g/ 0.9 oz)

Wet ingredients:

1 cup pumpkin purée (you can make your own) (200 g / 7.1 oz)

6 large eggs, separated

1/2 cup butter, ghee or virgin coconut oil, melted (115 g / 4 oz)

20-30 drops liquid Stevia extract

melted coconut oil or ghee for greasing

Note: When looking for ingredients, try to get them in their most natural form (organic, without unnecessary additives).

Instructions

Preheat the oven to 175 °C/ 350 °F. Place all the dry ingredients - apart from the pumpkin seeds - into a bowl and combine well.

I make my own chia seed meal by blending it in a food

processor for just a few seconds until powdered. Keto Pumpkin Chia Muffins

Separate the egg whites from the egg yolks. Using a hand beater or electric mixer (I'm using a Kenwood mixer), whip up the egg whites until they create soft peaks. In another bowl, place the egg yolks, melted butter, pumpkin purée and stevia.

The butter should be melted and cooled (don't use hot). The pumpkin purée and egg yolks should be at room temperature. If you use them straight from the fridge, the butter will clump up. Keto Pumpkin Chia Muffins

Process until well combined and start adding the dry mixture - a tablespoon or two at a time while mixing. Keto Pumpkin Chia Muffins

Add about a quarter of the whipped egg whites and mix gently. Add the remaining egg whites and fold in the batter using slow setting on your mixer or using a spatula. Be careful not to deflate the egg whites and keep the batter as fluffy as you can. Keto Pumpkin Chia Muffins

Line a muffin tray with 12 medium muffin paper cups.. Grease each cup with a small amount of coconut oil or ghee. Spoon the batter into the paper cups and transfer into the oven. Alternatively, you can use a silicon muffin tray or silicon muffin cups. Keto Pumpkin Chia Muffins

Transfer into the oven and bake for 5 minutes. After 5 minutes, sprinkle with the pumpkin seeds. Place back in the oven and bake for another 30 minutes or until the tops are golden brown. Keto Pumpkin Chia Muffins

When done, remove from the oven and place on a cooling rack. Store at room temperature for 4-5 days. Place the remaining muffins in freezer bags and freeze for up to 3 months. Enjoy!

41. KT MOZZARELLA DOUGH BGLS

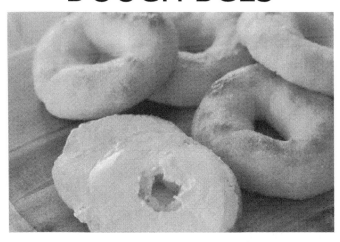

Prep Time: 10 mins

Cook Time: 15 mins

Total Time: 25 mins

Nutrition Facts:

Calories 203 - Calories from Fat - 151

Fat 16.8g - 26%

Carbohydrates 4g - 1%

Fiber 1.6g - 7%

Sugar 1g - 1%

Protein 11g - 22%

Ingredients

170 g pre shredded/grated cheese mozzarella

85 g almond meal/flour *see recipe notes below

2 tbsp cream cheese full fat

1 egg medium

1 tsp baking powder

pinch salt to taste

Instructions

Mix the shredded/grated cheese, almond flour/meal and cream cheese in a microwaveable bowl. Microwave on HIGH for 1 minute.

Stir then microwave on HIGH for another 30 seconds.

Add the egg, baking powder, salt, and any other flavourings, mix gently.

Divide the dough into 6 equal portions. Roll into balls then into cylinder shapes as shown in the video.

Fold the ends of the cylinder shapes in a circle and squeeze the two ends together to form a bagel shape.

Place on a baking tray and sprinkle with sesame seeds. Bake at 220C/425F for 15 minutes, or until golden brown.

42. KETO LW CARB NN BREAD

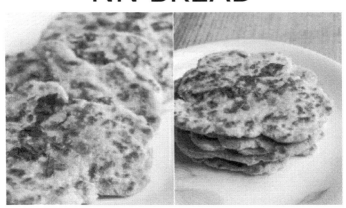

Prep Time: 10 minutes

Cook Time: 15 minutes

Total Time: 25 minutes

Nutrition Facts:

Calories - 370

Fat - 28g

Protein - 22g

Total Carbs - 9g

Net Carbs - 6g

Fiber - 3g

Sugar - 1g

Ingredients

1/2 cup Coconut flour

1.5 tbsp psyllium husk powder

2 tbsp coconut oil

1/4 tsp baking powder

1-1.5 cups hot water

1 Tbsp minced garlic (optional)

1/4 tsp Pink Himalayan Salt

Instructions

Combine the coconut flour, psyillium husk powder, baking powder, salt and coconut oil. Add the minced garlic to the mixture.

Add 1 cup of hot water to start and combine. Add more hot water if needed. If the consistency is too wet add more psyllium husk powder

Knead with your hands for a minute and let it sit in a bowl for 15 minutes.

Pull apart the dough into as big or as little balls as you'd like and roll out using some parchment paper and a rolling pin.

Heat a skillet to medium heat and add a naan to the heated skillet. Flip after a couple minutes (it will be brown on the other side), and cook until browned on both sides.

43. SURDUGH KETO BAGUETTES

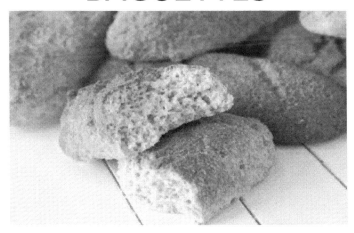

Prep Time: 10 minutes

Cook Time: 40 minutes

Total Time: 50 minutes

Nutrition Facts:

Calories 197 Calories from Fat - 90

Fat 10g - 15%

Carbohydrates 5g - 2%

Protein 14g - 28%

Dry ingredients:

  1 1/2 cup almond flour (150 g / 5.3 oz)

  1/3 cup psyllium husk powder (40 g / 1.4 oz)

  1/2 cup coconut flour (60 g / 2.1 oz)

  1/2 packed cup flax meal (75 g / 2.6 oz)

  1 tsp baking soda

  1 tsp salt (pink Himalayan or sea salt)

Wet ingredients:

  6 large egg whites

  2 large eggs

  3/4 cup low-fat buttermilk (180 g/ 6.5 oz) - full-fat would make them too heavy and they may not rise

  1/4 cup white wine vinegar or apple cider vinegar (60 ml/ 2 fl oz)

  1 cup lukewarm water (240 ml / 8 fl oz)

Tips:

Lukewarm water in this recipe will slow down the raising effect of baking soda. I tried both boiling water and lukewarm and although it made no difference for baguettes, some people have been experiencing air bubbles / hollow insides when making a loaf. More tips on the perfect loaf are listed here.

For a paleo, dairy-free option, try this coconut milk kefir recipe instead of the buttermilk: Use half of the coconut milk kefir and half water.

Make sure you use a kitchen scale for measuring all the dry ingredients. Using just cups may not be enough to achieve best results, especially in baked goods. Weights per cups and tablespoons may vary depending on the product/ brand or if you make you own ingredients (like flaxmeal from flaxseeds). Psyllium absorbs lots of water. When baking with psyllium, you must remember to drink enough water throughout the day to prevent constipation!

Instructions

Preheat the oven to 180 °C/ 360 °F (fan assisted). Use a kitchen scale to measure all the ingredients carefully. Mix all the dry ingredients in a bowl (almond flour, coconut flour, ground flaxseed, psyllium powder, baking soda, and salt).

Do not use whole psyllium husks - if you cannot find psyllium husk powder, use a blender or coffee grinder and process until fine. If you get already prepared psyllium husk powder, remember to weigh it before adding to the recipe. I used whole psyllium husks which I grinded myself. Do not use just measure cups - different products have different weights per cup! Sourdough Keto Baguettes

In a separate bowl, mix the eggs, egg whites and buttermilk.

The reason you shouldn't use only whole eggs is that the bread wouldn't rise with so many egg yolks in. Don't waste them - use them for making Homemade Mayo, Easy Hollandaise Sauce or Lemon Curd. For the same reason, use low-fat (not full-fat) buttermilk. Sourdough Keto Baguettes

Add the egg mixture and process well using a mixer until the dough is thick. Add vinegar and lukewarm water and process until well combined.

Sourdough Keto Baguettes

Do not over-process the dough. Using a spoon, make 8 regular or 16 mini baguettes and place them on a baking tray lined with parchment paper or a non-stick mat. They will rise, so make sure to leave some space between them. Optionally, score the baguettes diagonally and make 3-4 cuts. Sourdough Keto Baguettes

Place in the oven and cook for 10 minutes. Then, reduce the temperature to 150 °C/ 300 °F and bake for another 30-45 minutes (small baguettes will take less time to cook). Sourdough Keto Baguettes

Remove from the oven, let the tray cool down and place the baguettes on a rack to cool down to room temperature. Store them at room temperature if you plan to use them in the next couple of days or store in the freezer for up to 3 months.

Baked goods that use psyllium always result is slightly moist texture. If needed, cut the baguettes in half and place in a toaster or in the oven before serving. Sourdough Keto Baguettes

44. KETO PUMKIN BREAD FRNH TOAST

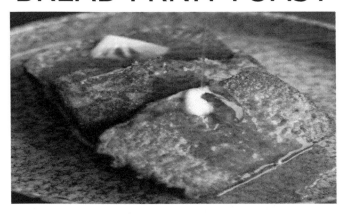

Prep Time: 10 minutes

Cook Time: 45 minutes

Total Time: 55 minutes

Nutrition Facts:

Calories: 165

Total Fat: 14g

Saturated Fat: 7g

Unsaturated Fat: 4g

Cholesterol: 99mg

Sodium: 76mg

Doc Julian

Carbohydrates: 6g

Fiber: 3g

Sugar: 1g

Protein: 5g

Ingredients

For the Pumpkin Bread:

  ¾ cup butter, melted

  4 large eggs

  1/4 cup unsweetened almond milk

  1 cup canned pumpkin puree

  2 cups almond flour

  1/3 cup coconut flour

  4 tsp baking powder

  ½ cup erythritol sweetener

  pinch of salt

  1 tsp ground cinnamon

  ¼ tsp ground nutmeg

  ¼ tsp ground allspice

For the french toast:

  2 eggs

  1/4 cup heavy whipping cream

  1/4 tsp ground cinnamon

  1 Tbsp erythritol sweetener

  8 slices pumpkin bread (3/4 inches thick)

1 Tbsp butter for frying

Instructions

For the pumpkin bread:

Preheat oven to 350 degrees (F)

Combine the melted butter, eggs, almond milk, and pumpkin puree in a blender and blend until smooth.

Combine the almond flour, coconut flour, sweetener, baking powder, salt, and spices in a medium bowl and stir well.

Pour the blender ingredients into the dry ingredients and stir until well combined and moisture is absorbed.

Line a long, narrow loaf pan with parchment paper and spoon the batter into a 12 x 4 loaf pan.

Bake the bread at 350 degrees (F) in the center of your oven for 60 minutes (or until a knife inserted in the center comes out clean.)

Turn off the oven and leave the bread in there for an additional 15 minutes.

Remove the bread from the oven and then from the pan using the parchment paper base to lift it out.

Cool on the counter or in the refrigerator loosely covered for a minimum of 4 hours, but for best results leave it overnight before slicing.

For the french toast:

Combine the eggs, heavy whipping cream, cinnamon and sweetener in a medium bowl and beat well until smooth.

Melt the butter in a nonstick saute pan over medium heat.

Carefully dip a slice of the pumpkin bread in the egg mixture on both sides for just a few seconds, and cook in the butter for about 2 minutes per side or until golden brown. Remove the french toast to a warmed plate and repeat with the remaining slices.

Serve warm with butter and sugar free syrup or cinnamon and sweetener sprinkled over the top.

45. 90 SECOND BREAD

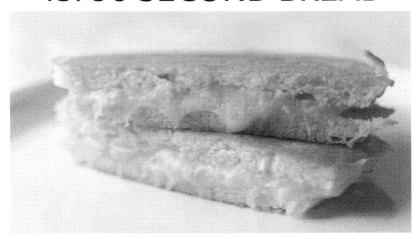

Prep Time: 3 minutes

Cook Time: 2 minutes

Total Time: 5 minutes

Nutrition Facts:

Calories: 235kcal

Carbohydrates: 5.7g

Protein: 8g

Fat: 20g

Fiber: 3g

Ingredients

    3 tbsp almond flour (or 1 1/3 tbsp coconut flour)

1 tbsp oil (melted butter, melted coconut oil, avocado oil)

1/2 tsp baking powder

1 large egg (See notes on how to make this less "eggy")

tiny pinch of salt

Instructions

Add all ingredients to a 4x4 microwave safe bowl, tap on the counter a few times to remove air bubbles, and microwave for 90 seconds. You can also bake in a oven safe container for 10 minutes at 375F

For 1 serving using almond flour: 315 calories / 29g fat / 4.7g carbs / 2g fiber / 11g protein

For 1 serving using coconut flour: 235 calories / 20g fat / 5.7 carbs / 3g fiber / 8g protein

To make this less eggy tasting, use just an egg white as the egg yolk is where the eggy taste comes from.

Tap the container on the counter a few times to remove any air bubbles before you cook it

You could really use any nut flour that you want if you are allergic to almonds or coconut. For alternative nut flours like pecan four, you would use 3 tbsp. You use half the amount for coconut flour because it's not really a nut and it is very absorbent!

I found that a 4x4 microwave safe container made the perfect size piece of low carb bread that could be cut in half and stuffed with all the things

You could also use a round container that is 4 inches in diameter for a keto mug bread

If you would rather bake this in the oven, you can use an oven safe container and bake at 375 for 10 minutes

Toasting this low carb bread makes it have a much better texture. you could also use a skillet to toast it in some butter.

46. KT FTHD BGLS

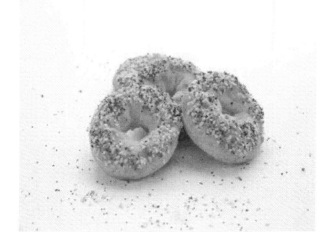

Prep Time: 20 mins

Cook Time : 20 mins

Total Time : 40 mins

Nutrition Facts:

Calories 190 Calories from Fat - 111

Fat 12.3g - 19%

Carbohydrates 5.5g - 2%

Fiber 2.6g - 10%

Protein 12.1g - 24%

Ingredients

    1/2 cup coconut flour (56g)

    2 tsp baking powder

    3/4 tsp xanthan gum

    12 oz pre-shredded part skim mozzarella

    2 large eggs

Optional Topping for Everything Bagels

    1 tsp sesame seeds

    1 tsp poppyseed

    1 tsp dried minced onion

    1/2 tsp coarse salt

    1 tbsp butter melted

Instructions

Preheat the oven to 350F and line a large baking sheet with a silicone liner. In a medium bowl, whisk together the coconut flour, baking powder, and xanthan gum. Set aside.

In a large microwave safe bowl, melt the cheese on high in 30 second increments until well melted and almost liquid. Stir in the flour mixture and the eggs and knead in the bowl using a rubber spatula.

Turn out onto the prepared baking sheet and continue to knead together until cohesive. Cut the dough in half and cut each half into 4 equal portions so that you have 8 equal pieces of dough.

Roll each portion out into a log about 8 inches long. Pinch

the ends of the log together.

In a shallow dish, stir together the sesame seeds, poppyseed, dried onion, and salt. Brush the top of each bagel with melted butter and dip firmly into the everything seasoning. Set back on the silicone mat.

Bake 15 to 20 minutes, until the bagels have risen and are golden brown.

47. KETO CHEESY BREADSTICKS

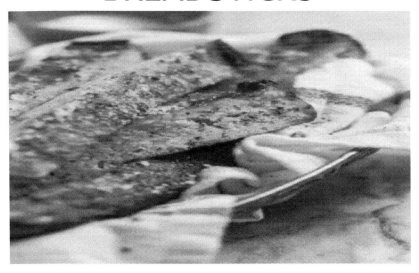

Prep Time: 20 minutes

Cook Time: 45 minutes

Total Time: 1 hour, 5 minutes

Nutrition Facts:

Total Fat 15.9g - 24%

Total Carbohydrate 4.6g - 2%

Dietary Fiber 0.9g - 4%

Protein 13g - 26%

Ingredients

Breadsticks:

4 eggs

1 ¼ cup (140g) shredded mozzarella cheese

¼ cup + 1 tbsp (37g) grated parmesan cheese

¼ cup (2 oz) unsalted butter, softened

1 oz cream cheese, softened

¼ cup + 1 tbsp (35g) coconut flour

1 ½ tsp Italian seasoning

½ tsp cream of tartar

½ tsp garlic powder

¼ tsp baking soda

¼ tsp salt

Topping:

2 cups (224g) shredded mozzarella cheese

¼ cup (30g) grated parmesan cheese

½ tsp Italian seasoning

Instructions

Breadsticks: Preheat oven to 350 degrees and coat 8×8 baking pan with nonstick cooking spray.

In a mixing bowl, using an electric mixer, mix together eggs, shredded mozzarella, grated parmesan, butter, and cream cheese until well-combined. Add coconut flour, Italian seasoning, cream of tartar, garlic powder, baking soda, and salt and mix again. Transfer mixture to prepared baking pan.

Topping: In a separate mixing bowl, mix together all ingredients until thoroughly incorporated. Sprinkle topping mixture atop breadstick dough in baking pan.

Final Steps: Transfer baking pan to middle oven rack and bake for 40 minutes. Then, turn oven broiler on and broil until topping is brown and bubbly, about 1-2 minutes. Remove pan from oven and allow breadsticks to cool before cutting into 10 pieces.

48. GARLIC PRMSN ZUCCHINI BREAD

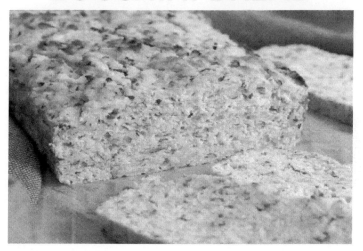

Prep Time: 20 minutes

Cook Time: 45 minutes

Total Time: 1 hour 5 minutes

Nutrition Facts:

Calories 112 - Calories from Fat - 50

Fat 5.6g - 9%

Saturated Fat 2.4g - 15%

Polyunsaturated Fat - 0.5g

Monounsaturated Fat - 1.3g

Cholesterol 61.6mg - 21%

Sodium 171.3mg - 7%

Carbohydrates 8.7g - 3%

Fiber 3.1g - 13%

Sugar 4.1g - 5%

Protein 8g - 16%

Vitamin A 200IU - 4%

Vitamin C 28.9mg - 35%

Calcium 200mg - 20%

Iron 1.4mg - 8%

Net Carbs 6g12%

Ingredients

4 packed cups shredded zucchini

3 large eggs

1 cup shredded parmesan cheese use a paleo parmesan dairy free cheese if you want to make it paleo

1 tbsp baking powder

1 tbsp garlic powder

1/4 cup superfine almond flour

6 tbsp coconut flour

Directions:

Preheat oven to 400°F. Line an 8 inch x 4 inch loaf pan with parchment paper.

Working in small batches, use a tea towel or several paper towels to squeeze water from zucchini. While zucchini does not need to be completely dried out, you want to eliminate

49. KT CINNMN SWIRL BRD

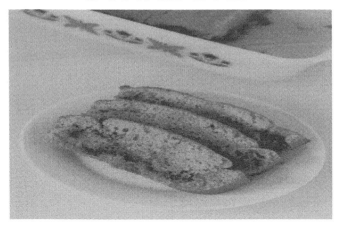

Prep Time: 15 minutes

Cook Time: 30 minutes

Total Time: 45 minutes

Nutrition Facts:

Calories: 161kcal

Carbohydrates: 3g

Protein: 5g

Fat: 15g

Saturated Fat: 6g

Cholesterol: 87mg

Sodium: 93mg

Potassium: 87mg

Fiber: 1g

Sugar: 1g

Vitamin A: 350IU

Calcium: 67mg

Iron: 0.8mg

Ingredients

- 4 eggs separated
- 1/4 tsp Cream of Tarter
- 2 tbsp butter melted
- 2 tbsp butter softened
- 1 tsp vanilla
- 3 oz cream cheese softened
- Liquid Stevia To Taste I used about 12 drops
- 1 tsp Baking Powder
- 1 cup Almond Flour
- 1 1/2 tsp Cinnamon divided
- 1/4 cup Erythritol I prefer confectioners

Instructions

Preheat the oven to 350 degrees F, and prepare a 9×5" loaf pan with non stick spray.

Separate the eggs into 2 large bowls.

Add the cream of tarter to the egg whites and beat with an

electric mixer until soft peaks form. Set aside.

Add softened butter, vanilla, cream cheese, and stevia to the egg yolks. Mix until well combined. Then add 1/2 tsp of cinnamon, baking powder and almond flour, stirring until well combined.

In a small bowl, combine the melted butter, erythritol, and the remaining 1 tsp of cinnamon. Stir to combine and set aside.

Fold the egg whites into the egg yolk mixture. This may take a few minutes as the egg yolk mixture may be fairly thick.

Pour half of the egg mixture into the prepared loaf pan. Evenly top with the cinnamon and butter mixture. Then the remaining egg mixture, ensuring that the mixture has been spread to the edges of the pan.

Using a butter knife, make swirls into the bread, keeping the knife vertical to prevent too much mixing between the layers.

Bake for 30-40 minutes or until the top is golden.

50. CHI PUMKIN BRD

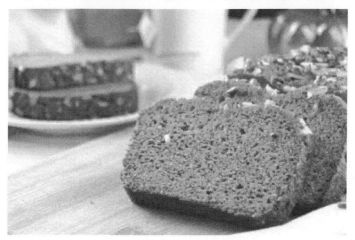

Prep Time : 10 mins

Cook Time : 45 mins

Total Time : 55 mins

Nutrition Facts:

Calories 190 - Calories from Fat - 126

Fat 14g - 22%

Saturated Fat 6g - 38%

Cholesterol 124mg - 41% Sodium 317mg - 14%

Potassium 303mg - 9%

Carbohydrates 9g - 3%

Fiber 4g - 17%

Sugar 1g - 1%

Protein 7g - 14%

Vitamin A 2460IU - 49%

Vitamin C 0.6mg - 1%

Calcium 148mg - 15%

Iron 1.5mg - 8%

Ingredients

8 eggs

1 cup almond flour

3/4 cup coconut flour

1/2 tsp salt

2/3 cup + 1. Tbsp pumpkin puree

1 1/2 tsp. baking powder

1/2 cup Lakanto Golden Monkfruit Sweetener

1 tsp. baking soda

1 tsp. vanilla extract

1 tsp. cinnamon

1/2 tsp. ground cardamom

1/4 tsp. ground allspice

1/2 tsp. ground ginger

1/4 tsp. ground cloves

1/4 tsp. black pepper

1/4 cup sour cream

5 Tbsp. butter melted

1 Tbsp. sunflower seeds optional

1 Tbsp. sliced almonds optional

Instructions

Preheat oven to 350 degrees. Grease or spray a 8-9" loaf pan and line with parchment.

 Using a stand mixer and a whisk attachment, whip eggs until light, foamy triple in volume. This can also be done with a handheld mixer but use a large bowl to prevent splatter!

If using a stand mixer, switch to paddle attachment. Add almond and coconut flours, salt, sweetener, baking powder, baking soda, pumpkin, and spices to eggs and mix on medium speed till combined, scraping down sides at least once. Add sour cream, melted butter, and extract to the batter and mix again till combined.

Spoon the batter evenly into the prepared loaf pan and smooth out the top. If desired, sprinkle almonds and sunflower seeds evenly over the top of the batter. Bake at 350 degrees for 45 minutes to an hour or until a tester comes out clean.

Half way through baking and cover loosely with foil to prevent over browning! If you use a 9" pan the baking time will be slightly shorter, so keep an eye on it starting at 30 minutes!

Cool in the pan. Using the parchment lift the loaf out of the pan and slice! Enjoy with a cup of coffee! This bread should be wrapped and stored in the fridge or it can be frozen whole or in slices.

CONCLUSION

Keto diets have really come on strong in the past year and a half and for good reason. It's a great way to not only shed those unwanted pounds quick, but also a great way to get healthy and stay that way. For those that have tried the Keto Diet and are still on it, it's more than just a diet.

It's a way of life, a completely new lifestyle. But like any major shift in our lives it is not an easy one, it takes an incredible amount of commitment and determination.

Although a ketogenic diet has been used to greatly improve people's quality of life, there are some out there who do not share the majority's way of thinking. But why is that exactly?

Ever since we can remember we have been taught that the only way to get rid of the extra weight was to quit eating the fat filled foods that we are so accustomed to eating every day.

So instructing people to eat healthy fats (The key word is Healthy) you can certainly understand why some people would be skeptical as to how and why you would eat more fat to achieve weight lost and achieve it fast. This concept goes against everything we have ever known about weight loss.

The ketogenic diet is high in fat, low in carbohydrates, and is designed to provide adequate protein and calories for a healthy weight. The essential aim of the diet is to prompt the body to burn fat instead of carbohydrate, which has the effect of fast weight loss.

The high fat content can cause surprise and concern in a health conscious society which associates 'fat' with 'bad.' However, good fats are healthy and necessary as part of a controlled and balanced diet.

High levels of carbohydrates, on the other hand, can cause a spike in blood sugar levels, which can lead to obesity and low energy levels. Part of the appeal is the ketogenic diet is its success in achieving fast weight loss, so it is ideal for those with many pounds to shed.

The diet excludes high carbohydrate foods such as starchy fruits and vegetables, bread, pasta and sugar, while increasing high fat foods such as cream and butter. A typical meal might include fish or chicken with green vegetables, followed by fruit with lots of cream. Breakfast might be bacon and eggs, a snack cheese with cucumber.

There are many variants of the diet which including more relaxed versions of the regime. The initial few days of a ketogenic diet involves the body adapting to a different way of eating, which can prompt a feeling of 'withdrawal'. This is no surprise as modern western diet and foods are heavy in starch and sugar.

Following this adaptation period, however, those eating a ketogenic diet begin to enjoy many benefits. In addition to fast weight loss, there are increased energy levels.

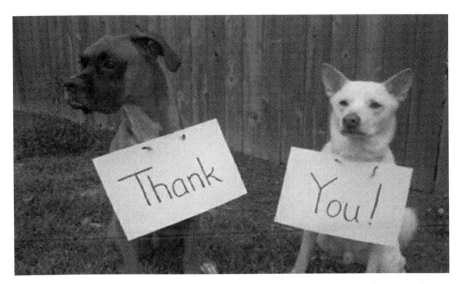

Finally, if you enjoyed this book, then I'd like to ask you for a favor, would you be kind enough to leave a review for this book on Amazon? It'd be greatly appreciated!

Click here to leave a review for this book on Amazon!

Thank you and good luck!

Made in the
USA
Columbia, SC